# Stressed Out

## About Difficult Patients

Joan Monchak Lorenz, MSN, APRN, BC

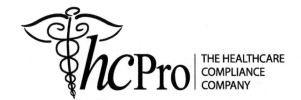

hcPro | THE HEALTHCARE
COMPLIANCE
COMPANY

*Stressed Out About Difficult Patients* is published by HCPro, Inc.

Copyright 2007 HCPro, Inc.

ISBN: 978-1-60146-012-7

Joan Monchak Lorenz, MSN, APRN, BC, Author       Audrey Doyle, Copyeditor
Michael Briddon, Editor                          Sada Preisch, Proofreader
Jamie Gisonde, Executive Editor                  Darren Kelly, Books Production Supervisor
Emily Sheahan, Group Publisher                   Susan Darbyshire, Art Director
Shane Katz, Cover Designer                        Claire Cloutier, Production Manager
Mike Mirabello, Senior Graphic Artist            Jean St. Pierre, Director of Operations
Michael Roberto, Layout Artist

Arrangements can be made for quantity discounts. For more information, contact:

HCPro, Inc.
P.O. Box 1168
Marblehead, MA 01945
Telephone: 800/650-6787 or 781/639-1872
Fax: 781/639-2982
E-mail: *customerservice@hcpro.com*

**Visit the Stressed Out Nurses Web site at: *www.stressedoutnurses.com***

08/2007
21271

# Dedication

I dedicate this book to its readers, who continually strive each day to enhance their nursing practice so they can provide quality care to the patients they serve.

# Contents

# Part II: Time for action

# Part III: Time for you

# How to use this book

What if there was a book that explained complex nursing topics in an easy-to-understand manner and in an accessible format? That's the premise behind the *Stressed Out…series*. Solid references with a bit of a sense of humor and the understanding that a lighthearted approach to learning makes the whole thing more enjoyable.

To help you navigate through the book, you will find the following icons highlighting a particular passage:

 **Don't forget:** A little reminder about something of importance.

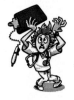 **Don't panic:** Take a deep breath and relax. Get ready for a little reassurance.

 **Fact:** Highlights a statistic or truth.

 **Tip:** A bit of inside information, a hint, or helpful advice.

 **Watch out:** Word to the wise; this is a warning.

**Listen up:** Powerful examples where effective communication leads to positive change.

 **Alarm:** An instance where poor communication can create dangerous or unhealthy situations.

**Happy Nursing! Now you're ready to get started.**

# About the author

## Joan Monchak Lorenz, MSN, APRN, BC

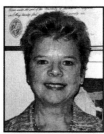 **Joan Monchak Lorenz, MSN, APRN, BC,** is currently working full-time as a member of the Nursing Education department of the Bay Pines VA Healthcare System, in Bay Pines, Florida. In this capacity, she works on hospitalwide educational initiatives for the nursing staff, as well as provides unit-based inservices and consultation on a variety of professional issues.

Joan has enjoyed a varied and well-rounded nursing career with clinical experience on both medical-surgical and psychiatric units. Her entrepreneurial nursing experiences include the founding of Hygeia, Inc., which provided psychiatric/mental health liaison and consultation services to individuals, healthcare facilities, and municipalities, as well as life-enhancing workshops for groups. She is currently the president of Clearly Stated, writing and editing health-related materials for healthcare professionals and the general public.

Throughout her career, Joan has cultivated an appreciation for cultural competency, having written and taught courses on issues related to cultural competency, as well as living and working in interior Mexico for a portion of three summers.

Joan has taught in a variety of nursing programs and continually reminds herself and others that nurses continually need to learn, as healthcare information has the habit of changing minute-to-minute.

Joan is a graduate from the Johns Hopkins School of Nursing and the Yale University School of Nursing. She is certified as an Editor/Writer and as an Educator by the American Medical Writers Association. Joan is board certified by the American Nurses Credentialing Center (ANCC) in Adult Psychiatric Mental Health Nursing.

# Acknowledgments

I want to thank those who have helped make this book a reality, with special thanks to my family, particularly my husband, Laird, for his patience and willingness to be benignly neglected on the weekends as I sat quietly in the office researching and writing this book.

I would also like to express my appreciation for the kind support and guidance given to me by Michael Briddon, editor of the *Stressed Out* series.

# Introduction

In jobs across the nation, nurses spend their days working with people—people who are scared, people who are sick or injured, people who need to make lifestyle changes to maintain their health, people who are caring for loved ones who are terminally ill, and people who are faced with making difficult decisions for either themselves or others. Even individuals who come to nurses because of a happy event—the birth of a baby, or the need for routine or preventive care—may be uncomfortable and uneasy when seeking care. They all have one thing in common: They are under stress.

Every nurse is taught that when people are under stress, they may not be on their best behavior. And this, in turn, causes stress for the nurse each working day. Being able to cope with the challenges of understanding behavior and of handling challenging situations is an area at the heart and soul of your nursing practice. Without it, all the technical skill and knowledge can be for naught. There is a continual need for exploration by each nurse every day.

## "Why is this person acting this way?"

How many times have you wondered what causes people to act in certain ways? And how many times have you said "if only"? If only he would cooperate more with the treatment . . . if only she would stay in bed and elevate her leg . . . if only he would stop throwing things across the room . . . if only she would pay attention to what I am saying . . . if only she would stop talking long enough for me to help her . . . if only he would keep his focus . . . if only she would quit flirting with the young doctors . . . if only . . .

If only the patient would do what he or she is supposed to do, healing would occur, and nurses could accomplish their goals of quality patient care. So, what keeps people from cooperating fully?

Let's find out. Let's start on this journey together. Let's shine some light on challenging behaviors and the conditions that cause them. Let's investigate the mystery of brain functioning. Let's put the puzzle together so that people with challenging behaviors can be understood and not shunned. Let's denounce the view of mental illness as a haphazard, confusing, erratic mess of impossible-to-understand disorders. Then, let's take a look at ourselves and see how we might change our point of view, our approach, and our responses to help make challenging patient situations easier to handle.

When the puzzle is put together, we will have a clear picture of why people behave in the ways they do, and how we can handle these unpleasant situations so that everyone is acting in the best way possible.

# Part One

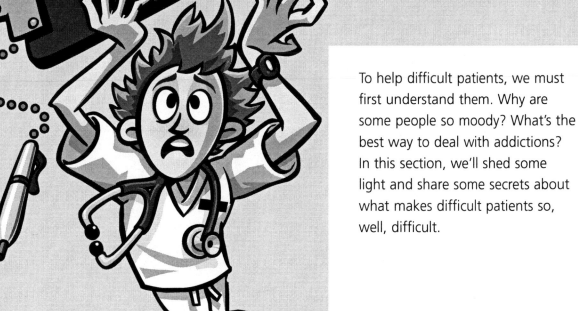

To help difficult patients, we must first understand them. Why are some people so moody? What's the best way to deal with addictions? In this section, we'll shed some light and share some secrets about what makes difficult patients so, well, difficult.

# Chapter 1

# Why do people act the way they do?

Before we get into the difficult behaviors of our patients, let's do a quick review of the brain. Understanding the way our brain processes information helps us understand why some people act the way they do.

## A brief review of brain function

Although the brain makes up only 2% of our body weight, it consumes 20% of the oxygen we breathe and 20% of the energy we take in. It controls everything we experience, including our movement and our ability to sense our environment, and regulates our body processes.

The basic functional unit of the brain, the **neuron**, connects with other neurons, sensory receptors, and muscle cells. A typical neuron has four structurally and functionally defined regions: the cell body, **dendrites**, **axons**, and axon terminals.

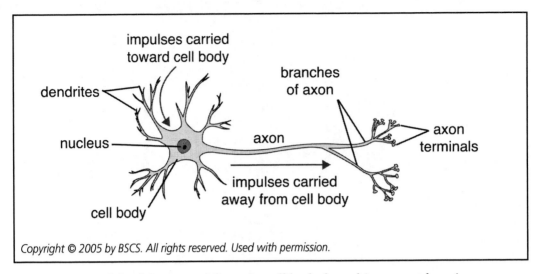

Neuronal **dendrites** extend from the cell body, branching out and serving as the main apparatus for **receiving** input from other nerve cells.

The neuronal **axon** carries messages away from the cell body, relaying these messages to other cells. Near its end, the axon divides into many fine branches that have specialized swellings called **axon terminals** or **presynaptic terminals**, which end near the dendrites of another neuron. The dendrites of one neuron receive the messages sent from the axon terminals of another neuron at the **synapse**.

The synapse is not a physical connection between the two neurons, but rather an electrical/chemical interchange in the intercellular space between the presynaptic neuron (the cell that sends out information) and the post-synaptic neuron (the cell that receives the information).

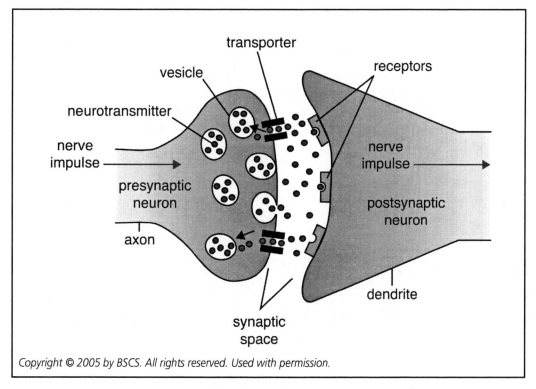

transporter

vesicle

receptors

neurotransmitter

nerve impulse →

nerve impulse →

presynaptic neuron

postsynaptic neuron

axon

dendrite

synaptic space

Neurons relay their information using both electrical signals and chemical messages in a process called neurotransmission.

Here's how the interchange at the synaptic space works:

1. An electrical impulse is carried away from the neuron along the axon of the presynaptic neuron.

2. When it reaches the presynaptic axon terminal, the electrical signal triggers the release of chemicals (neurotransmitters) that cross the synapse to affect the postsynaptic cell.

3. The neurotransmitters drift across the synaptic cleft and bind to special proteins (receptors) on the postsynaptic neuron.

4. An electrical impulse is generated that moves away from the dendrite toward the cell body.

5. Specific proteins (transporters or reuptake pumps) carry the neurotransmitters back into the presynaptic neuron, to await the next electrical impulse to reach the axon terminal.

6. Enzymes present in the synaptic space degrade neurotransmitter molecules that are not taken back up into the presynaptic neuron.

Each neuron specializes in the synthesis and secretion of a single type of neurotransmitter. Some of the predominant neurotransmitters in the brain include glutamate, gamma-aminobutyric acid, serotonin, dopamine, and norepinephrine. Each of these neurotransmitters has a specific distribution and function in the brain.

Many of the behaviors attributed to mental illnesses are most likely the result of problems with neurotransmission:

- **Depression and serotonin:** For example, serotonin levels are lower in individuals who have depression. Thus, the medications commonly used to treat depression—specifically, selective serotonin reuptake inhibitors (SSRIs)—relieve the symptoms by reducing the amount of serotonin that is taken back into the presynaptic neuron, leading to an increase in the amount of serotonin available in the synaptic space for binding to the receptor on the postsynaptic neuron.

- **Schizophrenia and dopamine, glutamate, and norepinephrine:** On the other hand, disruptions in the neurotransmitters dopamine, glutamate, and norepinephrine are common in individuals with schizophrenia.

So, simply put, one reason people behave the way they do is often a direct result of brain functioning.

## References

"Information about Mental Illness and the Brain." The Science of Mental Illness. Available at *http://science-education.nih.gov/supplements/nih5/Mental/guide/info-mental-a.htm*. Accessed June 2, 2007.

# Chapter 2

# Obstacles to
# good behavior

Besides neurotransmission problems in the brain, other issues can cause people to behave in unexpected ways. These issues fall under three categories:

- A lack of understanding

- An inability to comprehend

- An unwillingness to participate

## Obstacle 1: A lack of understanding

Sometimes a person's challenging behavior is due simply to a lack of understanding. The person just doesn't get it. Even adults who are confident and secure in other parts of their lives may feel insecure upon entering a healthcare facility. This holds true for our patients, the parents of children who are our patients, and adult children of our aging patients.

It is fairly common for people to misinterpret something someone said or did. This is more likely to happen when people are in an environment that is unfamiliar to them, an environment they might find intimidating.

Imagine going to a foreign country, a country with a culture very different from what you encounter each day, a country where no one speaks your language. You may be bewildered. You hear words that have no meaning to you; the tempo and the rhythm of the place are not ones in which you are familiar; and the people around you look the same as you in some aspects but not in others. In short, you are bombarded by newness at every turn. Many of us in this situation have experienced what is referred to as **culture shock**: anxiety produced when a person moves into a completely new environment. Culture shock is defined as "not having a sense of direction, the feeling of not knowing what to do or how to do things in a new environment, and not knowing what is appropriate or inappropriate" (Guanipa).

Why do people feel intimidated when entering a healthcare facility? Why is it so hard to understand healthcare professionals? Because just like in the preceding example, these people have entered a different culture: the healthcare culture.

Nurses work in healthcare facilities every day. We are used to the language, the pace, and the environment. We are so accustomed to the situations around us that many of us no longer even pay attention to the noises, the smells, and the particular attributes of the setting.

**Alarm:** Pam, a nurse, took her husband to a local ED for what turned out to be kidney stone pain. She felt comfortable enough in the ED. She stayed by her husband and helped him as much as she could. However, she could tell that the other nurses did not see what she was seeing: They did not see the person picking up the trash within six inches of the young, emaciated woman trying to eat her breakfast. They did not see the open supplies cluttered on the desk. They did not see that when they walked between two patient cots in the hallway en route to the supply area, noisy squeaks were emitted each time the two swinging doors to the area were opened. They did not see that her husband had no privacy when asked to give a urine sample. They did not see her holding the blanket around him for privacy while he knelt on the stretcher to fill the urinal. They did not see how the clustering of staff members around the desk appeared to the patients. Why didn't they see these things? Because they were so accustomed to the noise, the tight spaces, the clutter, and the lack of privacy. It was their space, not Pam's or her husband's.

Many aspects of healthcare cause confusion for the seeker of healthcare. For some people, walking into a healthcare facility is like walking into a different country with a different culture. They may not know how to navigate this new culture. This disconnect and subsequent confusion negatively influence clear communication and understanding between healthcare providers and those receiving the healthcare.

First, there is the use of a foreign language. Often, medical jargon—strange words, acronyms, and abbreviations—can make our patients' heads spin. Then there is the setting: beds with buttons, levers, and cords; strange contraptions that beep and hum; lights that are too bright; and "routines" that are unfamiliar. In addition, one's privacy is invaded. People walk in and out of the patient's room each day, performing tasks around and to them. For many people, the constant bombardments of different people add considerable stress.

 **Don't forget:** It is important to keep in mind that our patients and their families may not understand us. Their inappropriate or difficult behaviors may be a sign of their confusion, lack of understanding, and/or frustration. And as a nurse, you may be the first to become aware of their frustration and culture shock.

## Obstacle 2: An inability to comprehend

Language differences are an obvious obstacle to a person's ability to comprehend information. However, there are other obstacles to comprehension. These include the inability to hear clearly, the inability to process information as quickly as it comes in, and other interferences in processing information, such as incorrect interpretation.

For example, patients with delirium or dementia often are not able to comprehend what is happening around them. When bombarded with too much stimuli, the person with cognitive impairment might lash out in frustration.

### The impact of stress on learning

Another obstacle to comprehension is stress. Whether stress helps or hinders learning is now being debated in research circles. Joels et al. noted that "on the one hand it is generally accepted that stressful events are very well remembered: the more salient, the better remembered. . . . Yet, stress has also been associated with impaired cognitive performance." More research is needed to determine what types of stress enhance learning and what types hinder it. Currently, the general consensus is that some stress congruent with the learning experience aids in learning, whereas unfocused stress hinders learning.

 **Don't forget:** For our purposes, it is important to recall that patients under stress and unable to concentrate are not the best candidates for understanding what is going on around them. So, it is always best for nurses to determine a person's stress level, level of ability to concentrate on what is being said, interest in the subject, and attention to the conversation before attempting to give him or her any type of instruction.

## Obstacle 3: An unwillingness to participate

A third obstacle is an unwillingness to cooperate or participate. Nurses need to determine why patients seem to be unwilling to do what is expected of them. Some people are just plain set against making any changes or adjustments in their lives. But others may be unwilling to cooperate for less obvious reasons. It is very important for you to differentiate between unwillingness and inability. Your first step is to assess the patient to make sure he or she is simply not able to do what is expected of him or her.

**Listen up:** Take a moment and talk with the patient about what is holding him or her back from doing what has been asked. What appears as simple unwillingness might actually be due to:

- Fear of failure

- Fear of the unknown

- Inability to see the connection between actions and change

- Inability to see the reason to change

- A need for the patient to have the idea him or herself

When the underlying issue is addressed, the patient may then become more of a partner in his or her care.

## References

Boekaerts, M. (2002). *Motivation to Learn*. International Academy of Education. International Bureau of Education. Education Practices Series #10. Available at *www.ibe.unesco.org/publications/EducationalPracticesSeriesPdf/prac10e.pdf*. Accessed June 8, 2006.

Guanipa, C. (1998). "Culture Shock." Available at *http://edweb.sdsu.edu/people/CGuanipa/cultshok.htm*. Accessed June 2, 2007.

Joels, M., Z. Pu, O. Wiegert, M. Oitzl, and J. Krugers (2006). "Learning under stress: How does it work?" *TRENDS in Cognitive Sciences*, 10(4):152–158.

Lorig, K., D. Sobel, A. Stewart, B. Brown Jr., P. Ritter, V. González, D. Laurent, and H. Holman (1999). "Evidence suggesting that a chronic disease self-management program can improve health status while reducing utilization and costs: A randomized trial." *Medical Care*, 37(1): 5–14.

# Chapter 3

# Handling psychotic symptoms

Many nurses have problems handling people who have strange and some-times scary behaviors. That is completely understandable. Any nurse would be troubled if he or she had to care for someone and felt ill-equipped to do so. A nurse would not opt to care for a patient on a ventilator without know-ing the workings of the ventilator. In the same way, a nurse caring for some-one who is experiencing psychosis needs to know how to handle the various symptoms of psychosis to feel comfortable caring for that person.

**Psychosis** is a generic psychiatric term for a mental state often described as involving a loss of contact with reality in conjunction with personality changes, causing deterioration in normal social functioning.

The term **delirium** is used to describe an acute psychotic state, with rapid onset, caused by an agent or condition that when removed or treated will result in the resolution of the psychotic state. An example of delirium is when a person hallucinates as a result of an atypical drug reaction.

Some argue that certain mental states that involve a loss of contact with reality are not really losses, but rather states on a continuum with normal consciousness.

Indeed, many of us have experienced altered states of consciousness. Maybe you have had strange experiences just before falling asleep or as you woke up. Many people have described hearing things or feeling like someone was present in the room with them. These **hypnagogic hallucinations**—unusual sensory experiences or thoughts that occur when a person is falling asleep— or **hypnopompic hallucinations**—unusual sensory experiences or thoughts that occur when waking up from sleep—are very common experiences.

**Alarm:** Rebecca, a nurse, recalls that she experienced an altered state of consciousness when reading the works of Carlos Castaneda, who describes his experiences living and studying with a Yaqui shaman. She was really getting into his books and experiencing his adventures as she read, sometimes to the point of overinvolvement. While reading his books one weekend, she became hypervigilant to happenings around her and became concerned that she may lose touch with reality. As she ate lunch with her friends, she explained to them what she was reading and how it was impacting her. She asked them to take her to the ED if she should become "crazy."

Some other conditions that cause psychotic symptoms include:

- Using recreational drugs, in particular, cocaine, amphetamines, and hallucinogens

- Withdrawal from certain drugs, such as alcohol and barbiturates

- Side effects of certain prescribed medications, including barbiturates, benzodiazepines, anticholinergics, atropine, antihistamines, and antidepressants

- Electrolyte disturbances, including hyper- and hypocalcemia, hyper- and hyponatremia, hypokalemia, hypomagnesemia, hypermagnesemia, and hypophosphatemia

- Physical conditions, such as brain tumors, epilepsy, serious infections, dementia with Lewy bodies, multiple sclerosis, Alzheimer's disease, and syphilis

- Severe stress, anxiety, or panic

- Disorders such as post-traumatic stress disorder and sexual trauma

- Certain types of seizures, and delirium tremens (DTs)

- Exposure to toxins, poisons, or lack of oxygen

- Sleep deprivation, usually lasting from four to six nights

- Overstimulation or severe manic episodes

## Making a definite diagnosis: Get to the bottom of it!

The first step in treating a person in a psychotic state is to determine the state's cause. Although you, as a nurse, are helping to prepare the patient for the necessary workup to determine the cause of the psychotic state, you can explain what is happening to help the patient focus and give direction to his or her part in the workup. Expect that the workup will include:

- Blood tests, including electrolytes, blood glucose, creatine phosphokinase (CPK), liver enzymes, ammonia levels, thyroid function, and vitamin B12

- Toxicology screen, urinalysis, and blood gas analysis

- Electroencephalograph, head CT scan, and head MRI scan

- Cerebrospinal fluid analysis and certain x-rays

### Give clear explanations

**Tip:** It is very important to explain procedures to the patient in words that the patient can understand. Do not use healthcare jargon when working with a person in a psychotic state.

For example, tell the patient that you need "to obtain a sample of his or her blood" and not that you need to "draw his or her blood." A psychotic patient may interpret you literally, become confused about why you need to draw a picture of his or her blood, and wonder what the needle, syringe, and tubes you are holding in your hand have to do with drawing a picture.

### Provide safety

Keeping the patient safe during the workup and the treatment process is also your responsibility as the nurse. The use of controlled environments such as quiet rooms or seclusion rooms may be needed. Using a seclusion room, or restraining a patient for a brief period, is always done for safety, not punishment. Indeed, some patients have found such procedures restful and therapeutically helpful.

## Getting the patient to participate in the care plan

During the workup and into the treatment of psychosis, always include the patient as a partner in his or her care. You need to determine how much involvement the patient can accept. Resist the urge to think that just because the patient is having psychotic symptoms, he or she is "totally out of it." Here is an example of how a patient with psychotic symptoms can still participate in treatment.

 **Listen up:** Sam, an outpatient, told his nurse he was having visual hallucinations of scary things but that he knew these things were not real, and thus was not afraid of them. It sounds a bit like a contradiction, but nonetheless, the patient was able to follow directions and participate in the workup and treatment plan.

Being able to differentiate and describe the symptoms of a psychotic state enables you to make a good assessment and look for resolution or progression of symptoms. Symptoms a patient may experience during a psychotic episode include:

- Hallucinations, or seeing, hearing, feeling, or otherwise perceiving things that are not perceived by others

- Delusional beliefs, or false fixed beliefs

- Disorganized thinking and speaking

- Extreme excitement and confusion

- Illusions, or mistaken perceptions

- A lack of insight into the unusual or bizarre nature of his or her behavior

- Problems with social interactions, and impairment in carrying out goal-directed activities

## A clearer picture of hallucinations and delusions

**Hallucinations** are perceived as real by the person having them, but not by others. Hallucinations come in many varieties, including auditory, visual, olfactory, gustatory, and tactile. Hearing voices is the most common type of hallucination, and the voices may include comments on behavior, orders to do things, and warnings of impending danger. Sometimes the voices talk with each other, usually about the patient.

Other types of hallucinations include seeing people or objects that are not there (visual hallucination) or smelling odors that no one else detects (olfactory hallucination). Olfactory hallucination may be a symptom of certain brain tumors. Patients also may feel things like invisible fingers touching

their bodies or bugs crawling on them (tactile hallucination). Tactile hallucinations are most common in other conditions such as DTs.

Some people in psychotic states, particularly those with schizophrenia, experience command hallucinations, or hallucinations telling them to do certain
things. Sometimes command hallucinations tell the patient that he or she is
no good and is worthless, and that he or she needs to harm him or herself
in some other way.

**Tip:** As a nurse, you need to ask patients whether they are experiencing
command hallucinations, and ensure that you prevent them from acting
on the commands.

**Delusions** are false personal beliefs that are not part of the person's culture
and do not change, even when other people present proof that the beliefs
are not true or logical. Some people's delusions are quite bizarre, such as
believing that their neighbors can control their behavior with magnetic
waves, that people on television are directing special messages to them, or
that radio stations are broadcasting their thoughts aloud to others.

- **Delusions of grandeur** occur when people think they are famous historical figures

- People with **paranoid delusions** believe others are deliberately cheat-
  ing on, harassing, poisoning, spying on, or plotting against them or the
  people they care about

Disorganized thinking and speaking can present in many ways. People with
disorganized thinking and speaking have difficulty organizing their thoughts
or connecting them logically. Speech may be garbled or hard to understand.
They may have "thought blocking," which is evident when a person stops
speaking abruptly, in the middle of a comment. When asked why he or she
has stopped speaking, the person may say that it felt as though the thought
had been taken out of his or her head.

Extreme excitement and confusion is evident by shifts in behavior, and loud,
disorganized speech and activity.

Illusions or mistaken perceptions can cause great confusion for the patient,
as well as for the nurse. Illusions can occur in unfamiliar settings for
almost anyone.

**Tip:** Check with your patient often and ask the patient whether he or she has any concerns about what is happening around him or her. Remember that people with paranoia take everything personally, and they may simply misinterpret a casual conversation between two nursing staff members as a plot against them.

Physical things such as shadows and alarms may be misinterpreted as well. It is always good to offer simple explanations of what is happening, or what has occurred that was unexpected. For example, if an alarm of some kind goes off, take the time to explain it rather than just letting it pass. This will relieve anxiety.

Lack of insight into the unusual or bizarre nature of the patient's behavior may cause frustration for the nurse, in that the patient does not perceive his or her behavior as being out of the ordinary.

Problems with social interaction and impairment in carrying out goal-directed activities require nursing intervention. Patients in psychotic states need regular prompting to complete their personal care and to maintain appropriate conduct. As a nurse, you are wise to stay close to them, giving gentle direction and providing encouragement to continue to perform needed activities, such as getting dressed or eating.

Specific treatment of signs and symptoms of psychosis varies depending on the cause of the psychosis. The goal of treatment is to control or reverse the cause of the psychotic symptoms.

**Tip:** As a nurse, provide a pleasant, comfortable, nonthreatening, and physically safe environment during the diagnosis and initial care phase of treatment when the patient is in the most distress.

## It's intervention time

In general, for each patient, make sure to do the following:

- Remove any toxins. If an obvious toxic substance is causing the symptoms, remove it. Stopping or changing medications may improve cognitive functioning even before treatment of the underlying disorder.

- Treat the condition contributing to the state. For example, treating the congestive heart failure or severe anemia will increase oxygen to the brain, or treating the underlying electrolyte imbalance will greatly improve mental functioning.

- Give medications to control aggressive or agitated behaviors, or behaviors that are dangerous to the person or to others. This will ensure safety. These medications are usually given in very low doses, with adjustment as required. Medications that may be considered for use include thiamine, sedatives, serotonin-affecting drugs (trazodone and buspirone), and dopamine blockers (such as haloperidol, olanzapine, Risperdal, and clozapine).

- Evaluate sensory functioning and provide for augmentation to senses as needed, by the use of hearing aids and glasses, for example.

Want more tips? Here are some general interventions to use when a person is in a psychotic state:

- Develop a trusting rapport with the patient. Use the patient's words to describe his or her experiences. Make nonjudgmental statements of acceptance.

- Make short but regular contact with the patient, always telling him or her when you will return.

- Approach the patient in a receptive and open manner.

- Approach the patient slowly and make eye contact. Do not demand that the patient make eye contact. Avoid eye contact yourself if it seems to be making the person suspicious. This helps reduce the possibility of the patient feeling threatened.

- Observe the patient for evidence that he or she is having auditory or visual hallucinations. You can tell this by observing the patient carrying on a conversation with no one else present or seeming to watch things that you do not see.

- Reduce stimuli and provide a quiet environment.

- Avoid arguing with the patient or trying to point out "reality." Instead, talk about the implied concern. For example, if a patient complains that a person was in his or her room all night rummaging around and keeping him or her awake, respond to the implied message by saying, "Gee, if I was awake and didn't get sleep, I would feel tired too." Respond even though you know no one had been in the room.

- Listen carefully and be patient. Don't rush the conversation. Make sure you understand what the patient is asking for. Repeat what you think he or she said. Or if you believe you can interpret what the patient wants, ask whether you are correct. For example: "Are you trying to tell me that you are thirsty?"

- Avoid touching the patient unless you know that this is okay with him or her.

- Give medication as ordered and wait until the medication takes effect before you try to teach or make any other interventions.

Still want more tips? Okay, keep these in mind when communicating with a person who is out of touch with reality:

- Get to the point. Keep communication brief, direct, and focused.

- Express yourself directly and specifically. Subtle clues (such as facial expressions) may be lost.

- Use praise effectively. The person may be painfully aware of his or her limitations.

- Speak in a calm, slow voice.

- Repeat, repeat, and repeat. Recall that the patient is distracted and disorganized and needs repetition to stay on task.

- Pay attention to your voice and avoid any hint of annoyance, or of feeling hurried or frustrated.

- Avoid standing too close to the patient.

- Remember that you can't out-argue psychotic symptoms. Do not try to talk the patient out of delusions or hallucinations. Reassure the patient of his or her safety. Tell the patient that you are here to help.

## Keep these hints handy

A person who is excited or disorganized for a prolonged period may experience an increased need for nutrients and fluids, and at the same time may not be aware that he or she is hungry. You may need to frequently offer high-calorie finger foods, and drinks with lids.

**Listen up:** Some people in psychotic states need to be reminded to go to the bathroom. Andrew, a young patient in a psychotic state, complained of severe lower abdominal pain. After a period of confused assessment, it was determined that the pain was from a full bladder. Remember to regularly ask the patient to take some time to go to the bathroom. Don't ask whether the patient needs to go; ask the patient to go, and then check that he or she went.

## Helping a person who is hallucinating

To help a person who is hallucinating:

- Always keep in mind that hallucinations are real to the person having them. Hallucinations can involve any of a person's senses (sight, hearing, taste, smell, and/or touch).

- Approach the person quietly while calling his or her name.

- Ask the person to tell you what is happening. Ask whether he or she is afraid. Determine the level of confusion.

- Talk with the person about the experience and ask what you can do to help.

- Suggest that the person tell the voices to go away.

- Distract the person or involve the person in other activities.

- Outsmart the hallucinations by providing alternative stimuli on which to focus, such as listening to music or watching TV.

- Do not hurry the person.

## Working with a paranoid or frightened individual

When working with someone who is frightened or paranoid:

- Don't argue. Find out what you can about the person's fears.

- Clarify any misconceptions if the person is receptive to listening to you.

- Use simple directions, if needed. For example, say, "Put the plate back on the table. No one here wants to harm you."

- Give the person enough personal space to prevent him or her from feeling trapped or surrounded. Remain quietly with the person.

- Move the person away from a noisy environment and into a quieter one.

- Help the person avoid the objects he or she fears. Walk with the person away from the feared situation.

- Ask the person to talk with you about his or her fears. Make a direct statement that you are not afraid.

- Focus the person on his or her immediate environment, rather than on his or her fear. Make reassuring statements, such as "I know you think the FBI is out to get you. You are in the hospital now and we have no FBI here."

- Tell the person everything you are going to do before you do it. Explain in words that the patient can understand.

- Remind the person that he or she is experiencing symptoms of illness and these will clear when the medications take effect. Offer medications that are prescribed by the person's health professional.

- Keep the lights turned on to help reduce misinterpretations of objects in the surroundings.

- Call for help if you think you, others, or the person is in danger.

## References

Mann, L., T. Wise, and L. Shay (1993). "A prospective study of psychiatry patients' attitudes toward the seclusion room experience." *General Hospital Psychiatry*, May, 15(3):177–182.

# Chapter 4

# Shining a light on schizophrenia

Many nurses feel ill-prepared when it comes to working with some of the most difficult patients: those who are chronically mentally ill. However, as with all others aspects of healthcare, each nurse's confidence increases as he or she learns more about the condition and what to do to help.

## Let's get the basics down

Without a doubt, the most misunderstood psychiatric diagnosis is schizophrenia. And for good reason. People with schizophrenia present in many different ways. And over the years, theories have been promoted that blame the disease on a variety of factors, including bad mothering and masturbation.

Indeed, schizophrenia troubles many health professionals. Hence, there is plenty of research on its etiology and treatment. One thing most healthcare professionals agree on is that schizophrenia is a chronic mental illness, with periods of remission and relapse.

Like other chronic illnesses, schizophrenia also has a wide range of severity—from mild forms in which individuals work and support themselves between infrequent relapses, to the most severe and debilitating forms, which cause individuals to spiral down into poverty and dependence.

Compliance with medication therapy has always been a concern in treating people with schizophrenia, leading to relapse and hospitalization. Medications to control the symptoms of schizophrenia also carry their own set of side effects, some of which are so disturbing that even with the medications, the person is unable to blend into the mainstream of society. And even with what is considered good medication control of symptoms, some patients with schizophrenia continue to have prominent symptoms that interfere with their ability to be totally independent.

**Tip:** Using correct terminology can help keep things clear. For example, crazy can mean a multitude of things—anything from madness and insanity, to wild enthusiasm (the crowd went crazy), to some degree of fondness (he was crazy about her). Insane is really a legal term meaning that the person has a mental illness of such a severe nature that he or she cannot distinguish fantasy from reality, cannot conduct his or her affairs, or is subject to uncontrollable impulsive behavior. Most nurses prefer to use diagnostic or descriptive terms to describe their patients rather than general, often overused terms, such as crazy and insane.

**Watch out:** Other conditions may be confused with schizophrenia. These are often called schizophrenic-like conditions and include:

- **Schizotypal personality disorder**, described as when a person has difficulty developing close relationships with other people, and may have delusions and other unusual behaviors

- **Schizoid personality disorder**, described as when a person appears aloof and displays little or no emotion

- **Schizoaffective disorder**, described as when a person has the symptoms of schizophrenia combined with symptoms of either mania or depression or both

## How do you know whether it's schizophrenia?

Influenced by classic films such as *The Three Faces of Eve* and *Sybil*, many people often confuse schizophrenia with multiple personality disorder (or split personality). Others perhaps remember Hannah Green's novel, *I Never Promised You a Rose Garden*, in which the writer describes her life as a young mentally ill patient. Later reviews of her symptoms reveal that she most likely did not have schizophrenia, a term used to describe a multiple of thought disorders during that time, but rather another mental illness, perhaps hysteria or depression.

**Don't forget:**

- Schizophrenia is not multiple personality disorder or split personality

- Schizophrenia is not caused by bad parenting or lack of care during infancy

- Schizophrenia is not due to personal weakness, laziness, or masturbation

- Schizophrenia is not the result of severe poverty or other socioeconomic hardships

We know that schizophrenia is a neuropsychiatric condition, that is, a disorder of the brain. It is both a thought disorder and an emotional disorder. What we don't know is exactly how the brain is affected. It seems to be a complex issue with many variables. Some theories of the etiology of schizophrenia include a genetic vulnerability, impaired mechanics of synaptic transmission, malfunctioning neurotransmitters, and differences in brain size and structure. Issues in the person's environment may also contribute to the development of schizophrenia. The condition is most likely caused by a combination of structural and functional brain anomalies, with environmental factors impacting the presentation of symptoms.

**Fact:** Schizophrenia affects approximately 1% of the population, or 2.4 million U.S. adults. Men and women are equally affected. The illness usually emerges in young people in their teens or twenties (Schizophrenia, NIMH).

Although children over the age of five can develop schizophrenia, it is rare before the teen years. In children, the disease usually develops gradually and is often preceded by developmental delays in motor or speech development. Childhood-onset schizophrenia tends to be harder to treat and has a less favorable prognosis than does the adult-onset form.

Several studies suggest that an imbalance of chemical neurotransmitter systems of the brain, including the dopamine, gamma-aminobutyric acid, glutamate, and norepinephrine neurotransmitter systems, are involved in the development of schizophrenia.

Family, twin, and adoption studies support the idea that genetics play an important role in the illness. For example, children of people with schizophrenia are 13 times more likely, and identical twins are 48 times more likely, to develop the illness than are people in the general population (Numbers, NIMH).

Imaging studies have revealed differences in brain structure and function in individuals with schizophrenia compared with control individuals. These changes include a reduced total volume of the cerebrum, a reduced amount of gray matter, and enlarged brain ventricles. Positron emission tomography, or PET, scans of identical twins have revealed that the twin with schizophrenia has lower brain activity in the frontal lobes than does the twin who does not have schizophrenia.

## Living with the illness

Schizophrenia affects all aspects of a person's life. Even though specific symptoms may vary, all people with schizophrenia have a few things in common. They have:

- Confused and disorganized thoughts, including the presence of delusions and hallucinations

- Problems expressing their feelings appropriately, and wildly bizarre, erratic, and unpredictable behavior

- Problems with personal relationships and the ability to relate to other people in meaningful ways

The subtypes of schizophrenia include:

- **Paranoid,** with preoccupation with one or more delusions and frequent auditory hallucinations

- **Disorganized,** with disorganized speech and behavior, and a flat or inappropriate (for the occasion) affect

- **Catatonic,** with stupor, extreme negativism, and peculiar involuntary movements

## Give it some thought

People with schizophrenia have atypical thought patterns and thought content for their culture and circumstances. They do not process information the same way that other people do. They often misunderstand their own treatment, and they are prone to misinterpret what is said and done to them during treatment. There may be a link between schizophrenia brain functioning and language processing, meaning that people with schizophrenia may not be able to process language in the same way that others do. The brain is just not functioning in a way that makes thoughts and language coincide. Thus, people with schizophrenia may not be able to clearly articulate their thoughts through words.

Remember that in most people there is a direct link between what a person says and what a person is thinking. The thought occurs in the brain, and is then expressed through words. So what you hear from the person's mouth is a snapshot of what is going on in the person's thoughts. The thoughts and words of a person with schizophrenia may not be linked in such a direct way, and thus there is a disconnect between the person's thoughts and verbalizations. That may explain why the person is sometimes thought of as talking in a personal and mysterious language.

 **Tip:** Here are some ways that schizophrenic thought processes are expressed:

- Concrete thinking: interpreting things exactly as they are said

- Neologism: making up words

- Clang speech: rhyming all words spoken

- Word salad: stringing words together that make no sense

- Echolalia: repeating exactly what someone else has said

- Echopraxia: repeating exactly what someone else has done

- Perseveration: repeating the same activity (word or behavior) over and over again

So, what can you do? Here are a few hints to help you develop rapport with people who are not clearly articulating their thoughts:

- Observe their nonverbal communication, that is, their facial expressions and physical behaviors. What might these be telling you about their state of mind? Are they huddled in the corner and appear timid and unable to approach you? Are they pacing and looking increasingly frustrated and agitated? These mannerisms can give you a lot of information to help you know how to approach people. Take action to provide them with the care they need depending on their nonverbal presentation. If possible, check out your observations with them.

- Observe their language. What is the *feeling tone* behind the words they are using? Are they using sad and hopeless words? Scary and terrifying words? Look beyond the words themselves to the feeling tone of the words to discern their message. Then, check out your observations with patients to see whether you have interpreted their feelings correctly.

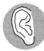

**Listen up:** Luke, a registered nurse who was spending time over a period of days with one very ill patient with schizophrenia at a state facility, made a very astute observation. He noted that each time the patient was scheduled for an appointment with his therapist, he could be found sitting in the day room, staring out the window, complaining that there was a "man sitting on top of the flagpole outside with a machine gun." He explained that this man was out to get him. After observing this behavior on a number of occasions, Luke looked beyond the words to the feeling tone, and hypothesized that perhaps the patient was using symbolic language to express his concern about his upcoming appointment. Luke surmised that the man with the machine gun sitting on the flagpole was the therapist, sitting high in the air to denote that he had more power and prestige than the patient, and he had something that he could use to harm the patient (the gun). Luke talked with the patient using his "symbolic language" to explore the patient's fear of the therapist, and in doing so was able to help the patient express his fears, and eventually help him relax before going to his appointment.

### Problems expressing emotions

People with schizophrenia may not be able to express emotion, or they express emotions that are inappropriate for the situation. They may experience:

- Depersonalization, or feeling unreal

- Ambivalence, or having conflicting feelings about people, things, or events

- Regression to earlier stages of development

## Signs and symptoms

Positive signs/symptoms are things we can observe. They include unusual thoughts or perceptions, including hallucinations, delusions, unusual thought processes, and disorders of movement. Chapter 3 discussed interventions to handle these behaviors.

Negative signs/symptoms are things that the person lacks. They include an inability to initiate plans, speak, express emotion, or find pleasure in everyday life. These signs/symptoms are often continually present and can be mistaken for laziness or depression. Assessing symptom presence and setting realistic goals comes with practice. Negative signs of schizophrenia include:

- Flat or blunted affect: not expressing emotions or expressing them inappropriately.

- Alogia: not talking or talking only with short statements. Alogia is not the same as refusing to talk.

- Avolition: not starting or completing tasks on one's own.

- Anhedonia: not being able to enjoy pleasurable things.

Patients with schizophrenia often also have other cognitive deficits such as problems with attention, certain types of memory, and the executive functions that allow us to plan and organize. The negative signs/symptoms of schizophrenia and the cognitive deficits are very disabling in terms of leading a normal life.

When people with chronic mental illness are hospitalized, they are often unkempt, malnourished, and in need of medication for stabilization. Nurses might have trouble getting past their appearance. But getting past their appearance is exactly what you need to do. If you view their appearance as a consequence of their symptoms, that is, avolition, or the inability to begin or complete tasks on their own, it changes the scenario from one of rejection to one of compassion. Just like any other "dirty" or "contaminated" patient situation, gown and glove up, and get to work. Granted, sometimes a patient is not willing to accept such close contact and you may need to wait for the patient's medications to help him or her come around.

 **Listen up:** Sally and Jake got the reputation of being the personal hygiene masters of the unit. The two developed a way to bathe, shampoo, lotion, and nurture those who had been on the streets for many days. Is there a Sally or Jake at your facility? Are you one of them?

Tom Hanks' character in the movie *Cast Away* is a great example of how a person can look so bad after a long time without adequate personal hygiene. Perhaps you can view your chronically ill patients upon admission as castaways, or refugees, who have spent many days and nights wandering about trying to find their way home. You, as their caregiver, have the opportunity to help them "get cleaned up real good."

**Tip:** Here are some other interventions for handling the negative signs/symptoms of schizophrenia:

- Offer hope and genuine emotional support: understanding, patience, affection, and encouragement.

- Refrain from showing frustration, or trying to hurry the patient.

- Engage the person in conversation and listen carefully.

- Gently encourage the patient to do some things for him or herself.

- Encourage participation in movement. Encourage participation in some activities.

- Set realistic goals. Do not push the person to undertake too much too soon.

- Balance the need for diversion and company with the need for a quiet environment.

- Break large tasks into small ones, and offer gentle encouragement to complete the tasks.

## Strange behaviors

People with schizophrenia display a multitude of movement and behavior disorders. These may include bizarre, erratic, and unpredictable behavior; talking out loud either to themselves or to active auditory hallucinations; and pacing, rocking, and repeating certain motions over and over. Most of the time, there is not much that can be done about these behaviors. Some will subside in time as the medication begins to take effect. Other behaviors will remain, and the nurse's role may include helping the person live with them and find ways to conceal or mask them.

### Other conditions that also can occur in people with schizophrenia

Many people with schizophrenia are bothered by suicidal thoughts, often with command auditory hallucinations telling them to kill themselves because they are useless and worthless. This makes suicide the most serious complication of schizophrenia. As many as 55% of people with schizophrenia may try to kill themselves, with about 10% of them being successful (Numbers, NIMH). We will discuss handling suicidal behaviors in Chapter 17.

# References

"Schizophrenia." National Institute of Mental Health. Available at *www.nimh. nih.gov/healthinformation/schizophreniamenu.cfm*. Accessed June 2, 2007.

"The Numbers Count: Mental Disorders in America." National Institute of Mental Health. Available at *www.nimh.nih.gov/publicat/numbers.cfm*. Accessed June 2, 2007.

# Chapter 5

# Why are some people so moody?

All of us have felt sad and blue at one time or another in our lives. It can be a normal reaction to the stresses of life. It certainly is an expected reaction to loss, such as the death of a loved one. However, if the condition lasts for a long period and interferes with a person's well-being and ability to care for him or herself, it is more likely a treatable physical condition: depression.

Nurses rally around a particular patient or coworker who experiences a loss. But what happens when the person's crying and need for reassurance lasts for longer than two weeks? Or when a person is always negative, low on energy, irritable, and unable to have any fun? In short, how do you treat a downer or a wet blanket? Patients like this may be seen as annoying, demanding, and cranky. No one wants to care for them. Nursing staff members may be slow to answer their call lights. Nursing staff members may become frustrated with the same complaints being made over and over.

Depression has been called the common cold of mental illness. It can be highly contagious, sucking in others in its midst. People can be influenced by depression and not recognize it as depression. Some people live in depressed households and don't know of any other lifestyle. Negativity, physical illnesses, irritability, pessimism, rudeness, sarcasm, and the silent treatment can all be signs that depression has taken over a person's life.

The sooner you spot this creature the better, the sooner it is acknowledged as depression the better, and the quicker treatment is started the better.

Research proves that depression can be contagious. In 1994, Joiner reported on a study in which 96 pairs of college roommates were examined for the phenomenon of contagious depression during two assessment sessions separated by three weeks. Consistent with prediction, roommates of depressed target students became more depressed themselves over the course of the three-week study (Joiner).

The amount of emotional energy needed to keep one's own energy up when caring for depressed people is often underestimated.

**Listen up:** Nurse Molly recalls a period on a small psychiatric unit when the majority of the patients there were depressed. Depression became very contagious: Staff members noticed that it took them longer to complete routine nursing tasks, complained of minor annoyances, and began to bicker with each other. Because the staff members trusted each other and worked well together, they shared their observations and realized that they were picking up on the mood of the majority of their patients. Always using humor to work through challenging situations, one staff member suggested that they call the emergency department and request that the first manic patient to come through the door be admitted to their unit. After that, the staff was able to work up a plan to help them get through the gloom on their unit. The charge nurse talked with the sister unit's charge nurse and set up a schedule that allowed the staff to switch between the two units. Staff members from each unit took turns going to the other unit. This reduced the amount of time any one staff member spent with depressed patients. Spirits rose and the staff was able to get past the contagion of depression.

**Fact:** Depression, or depressive disorders, are a leading cause of disability in the United States. Nearly 14.8 million Americans over the age of 18 suffer from major depression. In any given one-year period, 6.7% of the population age 18 and older suffer from a depressive illness (Kessler, et al.)

Unfortunately, many depressed people do not seek help because they do not perceive their symptoms to be those of depression. Left undiagnosed and untreated, depression can worsen, lasting for years and causing untold suffering, and possibly even result in suicide. Many depressed people seek help from a healthcare provider for various physical conditions. With the focus on physical symptoms and not their root cause, there is usually a delay in diagnosis and a delay in treatment for the depression.

All nurses need a firm grasp of the etiology and treatment for depression. Recognition and early treatment can avoid some of the difficulty these patients may bring to any nursing unit.

## How do I know whether it's depression?

Depression is not:

- The same as a passing blue mood

- A sign of personal weakness

- A condition that can be willed or wished away

- A condition that can be cured by merely "pulling yourself together"

Depression is an illness that involves the body, mood, and thoughts. It affects the way a person eats and sleeps, the way one feels about oneself, and the way one thinks about things. Biochemically speaking, people with depression have less of the neurotransmitter serotonin released into the synaptic space than people who are not depressed. Serotonin is important for the transmission of nerve impulses at the synaptic cleft and when there is not enough serotonin, things slow down.

### Forms of depression

Dysthymia is a less severe form of depression, but it tends to be more chronic. People with dysthymia may not be as disabled as those who are depressed, but they definitely have problems functioning well and feeling good.

No doubt nurses work with and care for dysthymic people every day. A dysthymic coworker may be crabby and irritable. A dysthymic patient may take a gloom-and-doom approach to his or her role in his or her healthcare.

### Other physical causes of depression

Depression, like other mental illnesses, is thought to be caused by a combination of biological, environmental, and social factors. Genetic causes have been suggested from family studies that have shown that between 20% and 50% of children and adolescents with depression have a family history of depression and that children of depressed parents are more than three times as likely as children with nondepressed parents to experience a depressive disorder (NIMH).

Abnormal endocrine function, specifically of the hypothalamus or pituitary, may play a role in causing depression. Also, changes in brain activity, as shown through PET imaging studies, have been noted in depressed individuals: Brain activity in certain areas is substantially decreased, whereas activity in other brain regions is increased. PET imaging has also shown that depressed patients have lower neurotransmitter receptor binding potential in some areas of the brain.

### Risk factors for depression

The following are risk factors for depression:

- People who have low self-esteem, are pessimistic, or are prone to become overwhelmed by stress are prone to depression

- Chronic stress, multiple losses, and other life-changing events make people more prone to develop depression

Multiple physical insults also make a person more prone to develop depression. Depression most frequently seen in general hospitals may result from multiple surgeries, major health events such as a stroke or heart attack, and chronic illnesses such as cancer or Parkinson's disease. Hormonal disorders can also cause depressive illness.

**Watch out:** As a nurse, you need to be continually watchful for signs of depression in all individuals you care for and in all chronically ill patients.

## Diagnosis difficulties

Unfortunately, many healthcare providers are still not savvy when it comes to spotting clinical depression. How many times have you heard statements such as "But of course, anyone would be depressed if they just lost their child" or "Anyone would feel sad and blue under theses circumstances"? Or "He is just getting older. People get slower and don't have as much fun at his age. He is 70 years old. What do you expect?"

It is time to replace these statements with objective data collection and analysis for what the real diagnosis might be: clinical depression.

**Tip:** Don't fall into the trap of discounting symptoms: Make an objective assessment and then follow through. Advocate for the person if your concerns seem to be pushed aside when communicated to those who might prescribe a further workup and treatment plan.

Typical depression scenarios might include:

- A staff member who is always pessimistic: "That will never work here," or "We tried that five years ago and nothing happened"

- A patient who is demanding, requesting small things from the staff, or always on the call light

- A family member who finds fault in the care of his or her loved one, who complains that medication is 15 minutes late, the meal is not hot enough, there isn't enough ice in the water, and so on

- A child who cannot be comforted, who clings, or who has an inordinate number of physical complaints

- A charge nurse who believes that every day is a catastrophe, blowing things out of proportion or living his or her life in constant disappointment

- A friend who is always seeking reassurance

## Spotting the sadness

Look for these signs and symptoms of depression:

- Expressions of sadness, emptiness, hopelessness, worthlessness, pessimism, and/or guilt

- Changes in sleep: either not enough (insomnia) or too much (excessive sleep)

- Changes in appetite: either not enough with weight loss, or too much with weight gain

- Changes in energy level: either too much (restlessness, irritability, and anxiety) or too little (no energy, feeling fatigued, and feeling slowed down)

- Loss of enjoyment from things that were once pleasurable, including sex

- Difficulty concentrating and making decisions, and/or forgetfulness

- Somatic complaints: stomachache, recurrent headaches, body aches and pains

- Thoughts of death or suicide, or attempting suicide

### Depression differences and the sexes

**Fact:** Women experience depression about twice as often as men (NIMH).

Hormonal factors associated with the menstrual cycle, pregnancy, miscarriage, postpartum period, premenopause, and menopause may contribute to the increased rate of depression in women. Some women have depression as a part of severe premenstrual syndrome.

Many women are also particularly vulnerable to depression after the birth of a baby (postpartum depression). Just when everyone thinks the woman should be the happiest, life to her seems a drudgery and void of happiness. In her book *Down Came the Rain*, Brooke Shields talks about her bout with postpartum depression. Her problems first began when her daughter Rowan was born. She describes that she was unable to form a bond with her, and states that the infant felt like "a complete stranger to me." At her lowest point, she had thoughts of jumping from a window. Thanks to medication and talk therapy, Brooke was able to recover and develop a loving relationship with her baby.

**Fact:** About 6 million men in the United States are affected by depression (NIMH).

- Men are less likely to admit to depression and are less willing than women to seek help

- Men mask depression by using alcohol or drugs, or working excessively long hours

- Depression in men may be associated with an increased death rate from coronary heart disease

- Depression in men can manifest as irritability, anger, and discouragement

## Working with patients of all ages

Those of us who work with the young need to be aware that not all moodiness is a temporary "phase" of development:

- A depressed child may pretend to be sick, refuse to go to school, cling to a parent, or worry that the parent may die

- Older children may sulk, get into trouble at school, be negative, be grouchy, and feel misunderstood

### How about the elderly?

Don't fall into the trap of considering any change in mental status in an older person as part of the "normal aging process." Those older adults who are cranky, forgetful, or hard to work with may be depressed. Remember that most older people feel satisfied with their lives. It is not wise to dismiss what could be signs and symptoms of depression as a normal part of aging. Special considerations about depression in older adults include the following:

- Depression may manifest itself with physical symptoms

- Depressive symptoms may be side effects of medications

## Put a smile on someone's face

Appropriate treatment can help people who are depressed, and includes continual assessment. It's essential to monitor symptoms and a patient's response to medication.

### Handling expressions of negativity

In general, remind patients that their negative feelings and attitudes are symptoms of their condition, and that positive thinking will replace negative thinking as they respond to treatment and their mood lifts. By doing this, you are also acknowledging that you believe the person is depressed and is not faking it. In addition, this provides hope that things will get better.

 **Tip:** You can also:

- Offer genuine emotional support: understanding, patience, affection, and encouragement

- Engage the depressed person in conversation and listen carefully

- Point out realities and offer alternatives

- Be nonjudgmental and accepting, and offer genuine praise

### Changes in sleep

Whether the patient is sleeping too much or too little, the goal is to have him or her develop a regular sleep pattern. Turn to Chapter 15 for hints in helping all patients who have problems with sleep.

### Changes in appetite

Patients who are depressed may overeat or not eat enough. Providing opti-
mal fluids and food is challenging. It is best to help those who overeat to
pace themselves throughout the day and to try foods that are lower in
calories. For those who undereat, try to offer small, frequent meals of high-
energy foods. See Chapter 15 for more on eating.

### Changes in energy level

**Tip:** People with depression feel exhausted, worthless, helpless, and hopeless. They often feel like giving up. They need gentle encouragement. Here
are some things you can do to help them handle their low energy levels:

- Assume a reasonable amount of responsibility. Gently insist that the
  patient do some things for him or herself.

- Set realistic goals. Do not push the depressed person to undertake too
  much too soon.

- Balance the need for diversion and company with too many demands,
  as this may cause a sense of failure.

- Break large tasks into small ones. Set priorities, and ask the patient to
  do what he or she can.

Chapter 9 includes a discussion on how to handle restless, irritable, and
anxious behaviors in patients.

### Changes in enjoyment

**Tip:** Patients who suffer from depression may no longer feel enjoyment
from things that were once pleasurable. To help:

- Encourage participation in some activities that once gave pleasure,
  such as hobbies, sports, or religious or cultural activities

- Encourage participation in mild exercise, even if the patient does not feel
  totally into it

- Encourage the patient to surround him or herself with people so that he
  or she is not alone

### Changes in concentration and decision-making

**Tip:** When a patient experiences changes in concentration or decision-
making, advise him or her to:

- Postpone important decisions until the depression has lifted

- Discuss any significant transitions, such as a job change, or getting married or divorced, with someone who knows him or her well

### Somatic complaints: Aches and pains

Patients who are depressed also get other ailments. Don't assume that every physical concern is a somatic presentation of a patient's depression. Always investigate each complaint to be sure it does not have a treatable cause. Common physical complaints of those receiving antidepressant therapy are dry mouth, slow emptying of the stomach, and constipation. As a nurse, you need to provide preventive guidance, as well as treat any of these should they occur.

### Thoughts of death or suicide

Always ask a person with depression if he or she feels so bad that he or she has thoughts of hurting or killing him or herself. See Chapter 17 for a thorough discussion on working with patients who are suicidal. In general, you, as the nurse, need to ensure safety, and you must continually assess the patient for the presence of a thought disorder as well as the presence of suicidal ideation.

## Spread the medication information

You play a crucial role when patients are started on medications to treat depression. This can be a very trying time: The patient may be experiencing side effects of the medications before experiencing any positive relief of the depressed mood. Because of this, he or she may refuse to take medication or continually question its effectiveness.

Antidepressant medications used to treat depressive disorders come in three major families: selective serotonin reuptake inhibitors (SSRIs), tricyclics, and monoamine oxidase inhibitors (MAOIs). They work by impacting neurotransmitters such as dopamine and norepinephrine. Make sure the patient knows that:

- Antidepressant medications must be taken regularly for three to four weeks (in some cases, as long as eight weeks) before the full therapeutic effect occurs (NIMH).

- He or she needs to resist the urge to stop medication too soon. The patient may feel better and think he or she no longer needs the medication. Or the patient may think the medication isn't helping at all. It is important to keep taking medication until it has a chance to work.

- Once he or she feels better, it is important to continue the medication for at least four to nine months to prevent a recurrence of the depression.

- Antidepressant drugs are not habit-forming. However, some antidepressant medications must be stopped gradually to give the body time to adjust.

- Antidepressants have to be carefully monitored to see whether the correct dosage is being given.

- People who take MAOIs need to avoid certain foods that contain high levels of tyramine: aged cheeses, wines, and pickles, as well as medications such as decongestants. The interaction of tyramine with MAOIs can bring on a hypertensive crisis, a sharp increase in blood pressure that can lead to a stroke.

- Never mix prescribed medication with over-the-counter medications. Always consult with the prescribing healthcare provider.

- Some drugs, such as alcohol or recreational drugs, may reduce the effectiveness of antidepressants and need to be avoided. This includes wine, beer, and hard liquor.

- Antianxiety drugs or sedatives are not antidepressants.

- Stimulants, such as amphetamines, are not effective antidepressants (NIMH).

Continued assessment for suicide is important as medications are being introduced. Suicide becomes a problem when the depressive symptoms start to lift. Prior to that, the person may have had thoughts of suicide, but didn't have enough energy to act on them. However, as the patient's mood lifts and his or her energy returns, he or she now has the ability to formulate a plan and the energy to carry it out. Now more than ever, it is imperative to regularly assess the patient for suicidal ideation.

### What's the deal with St. John's wort?

St. John's wort (hypericum perforatum), an herb used extensively in the treatment of mild to moderate depression in Europe, has recently aroused interest in the United States. Indeed, in Germany, hypericum perforatum is used in the treatment of depression more than any other antidepressant.

The National Institutes of Health conducted a three-year study that included 336 patients with clinical depression of moderate severity. The patients were randomly assigned to an eight-week trial with one-third of patients receiving a uniform dose of St. John's wort; another third sertraline, a selective SSRI commonly prescribed for depression; and the final third a placebo. At the end of the first phase of the study, participants were measured on two scales, one for depression and one for overall functioning. There was no significant difference in rate of response for depression, but the scale for overall functioning was better for the antidepressant than for either the St. John's Wort or the placebo (NIMH).

## That's what (family and) friends are for

The support and involvement of family and friends can be crucial in helping someone who is depressed. It is especially helpful if family and friends encourage the patient to stick with treatment and practice the coping techniques and problem-solving skills he or she is learning during therapy. As a nurse, you can help family members of people with depression. Suggest that family members:

- Educate themselves and others about depression to help them understand what their loved one is experiencing.

- Help their loved one with depression to stick to his or her treatment plan. This means making sure that medicines are available if prescribed, attending therapy sessions with the person if needed, helping the person to make recommended lifestyle changes, and encouraging the person to follow up with the proper healthcare provider, especially if the treatment needs to be adjusted.

You can also offer suggestions for living with a depressed person that may make things easier for family members and more beneficial for the depressed person:

- Recall that hostility, rejection, and irritability can be signs of depression. Encourage family members not to take these behaviors personally.

- Encourage family members to make time for themselves and their own needs. Taking regular breaks from the depressed person will help the family members and the patient.

- Ask family members to consider getting involved with therapy, either alone or with the depressed person. Support groups might also be helpful.

## Thoughts on therapy

Many people are depressed because of negative self-talk, or talk they internalized from what was said to them as children. This negative inner dialogue is so much a part of the person that he or she doesn't recognize it as something that needs to be addressed. In addition to negative self-talk, many people simply find themselves in life situations for which they are ill-prepared. They do not know how to get out of them, or resolve the issues that surround them. Short-term talk therapy can come to their rescue. It can help people gain insight into and resolve problems through verbal exchange with the therapist, sometimes combined with homework assignments between sessions.

How can therapy help?

- Behavioral therapists help patients learn how to obtain more satisfaction and rewards through their own actions and how to unlearn the behavioral patterns that contribute to or result from their depression

- Interpersonal therapists focus on a patient's disturbed personal relationships that both cause and exacerbate the depression

- Cognitive/behavioral therapists help patients change the negative styles of thinking and behavior often associated with depression

- Psychodynamic therapists focus on resolving the patient's conflicted feelings

### Trying ECT

Electroconvulsive therapy (ECT) is useful, particularly for individuals whose depression is severe or life-threatening, for those who cannot take antidepressant medication, or when antidepressant medications do not effectively relieve the symptoms of depression.

You may have heard horror stories about ECT. In recent years, however, many changes have been made to the procedure to ease its administration. For example, a muscle relaxant to reduce the physical signs and symptoms of tonic-clonic seizure activity is given before treatment, and the procedure is done under brief anesthesia. Electrodes are placed at precise locations on the head to deliver electrical impulses. The stimulation causes a brief (about 30 seconds) seizure within the brain. The person receiving ECT does not consciously experience the electrical stimulus. For full therapeutic benefit, at least several sessions of ECT, typically given at the rate of three per week, are required (NIMH).

You may initially feel that putting an electric shock to the brain is barbaric. However, don't we shock a person's heart who has collapsed from a myocardial infarction? Isn't the placement of AED pads and the defibrillator shock taught in most CPR classes? You probably agree that this is a life-saving intervention. And likewise, for a very depressed person who has not been helped by antidepressant medication, ECT can be a life-saving intervention.

## References

"Depression." National Institute of Mental Health. Available at *www.nimh.nih.gov/publicat/depression.cfm#ptdep1*. Accessed June 2, 2007.

"Depression and Suicide in Children and Adolescents." Mental Health: A Report of the Surgeon General. Available at *www.surgeongeneral.gov/library/ mentalhealth/chapter3/sec5.html*. Accessed June 2, 2007.

"Information about Mental Illness and the Brain." The Science of Mental Illness. Available at *http://science-education.nih.gov/supplements/nih5/Mental/ guide/info-mental-b.htm*. Accessed June 2, 2007.

Joiner, T. "A test of interpersonal theory of depression in youth psychiatric inpatients." *Journal of Abnormal Psychology* (February 1999).

Kessler, R., W. Chiu, O. Demler, and E. Walters (2005). "Prevalence, severity, and comorbidity of twelve-month DSM-IV disorders in the National Comorbidity Survey Replication (NCS-R)." *Archives of General Psychiatry*, 62(6):617–27.

# Chapter 6

# High-octane energy

Mania or an elevated mood is hard to miss. People who are manic have lots to say; have lots of places to go; have a wealth of ideas to share; and just don't have enough time to explain all of their theories, schemes, and plans. Much like the Energizer Bunny, people with mania keep going and going, often after all of those around them have dropped with exhaustion, or walked away seeking quiet and solitude.

People with mania, especially those who have hypomania (a milder form of elevated mood and elation), love their episodes when they can say "I get so much done," "I become super creative," or "I am on the top of my game." An episode can go something like this:

> At first, when I'm high, it's tremendous . . . ideas are fast . . . like shooting stars you follow until brighter ones appear. All shyness disappears, the right words and gestures are suddenly there . . . uninteresting people and things become intensely interesting. Sensuality is pervasive. The desire to seduce and be seduced is irresistible. Your marrow is infused with unbelievable feelings of ease, power, well-being, omnipotence, euphoria. You can do anything . . .

But then things take a turn:

> The fast ideas become too fast and there are far too many of them. Overwhelming confusion replaces clarity . . . you stop keeping up with it—memory goes. Infectious humor ceases to amuse. Your friends become frightened. Everything is now against the grain. You are irritable, angry, frightened, uncontrollable, and trapped (Spearing).

And therein lies the problem: While in manic episodes, people deplete all of their own bodily reserves, and the reserves of others. Those caring for the manic person become exhausted themselves, generally depleting all of their emotional as well as physical energy reserves.

## Seductive and destructive

People who are depressed usually know something is wrong, and they don't like the way they feel. But it's different for people who are hypomanic or manic. They usually don't think anything is wrong. They wonder what is wrong with those around them.

Mania and hypomania can be seductive. People feel more energized, creative, and interesting. Who wouldn't like feeling like that? Who wouldn't like being able to get extraordinary amounts of work done? Who wouldn't like feeling elated, being lifted up by success or exaltation? So, what's the problem?

Manic episodes often turn destructive. People in manic episodes wipe out their bank accounts; lose their reputations in their communities as well as ruin their marriages because of increased sexual drive and sexual escapades; lose jobs because of their inability to concentrate, poor judgment, and intense behavior; get intertwined in legal problems because of uncontrolled behaviors, such as speeding and gambling; and create immense financial problems due to uncontrolled spending sprees. The life of a manic person is a whirlwind . . . and then the whirlwind stops, sometimes leading to deep depression or a psychotic state.

People in mania also isolate themselves from others. They may become reckless and volatile. They irritate those around them, scare off those who want to help them, and leave a path of emotional destruction that may be hard to repair.

Picking up the pieces after mood swings can be hard. The people they need most—especially their friends and family—may be angry with them or reluctant to help.

Most dangerous of all, mania can make people do things that risk their lives and/or the lives of others.

**Tip:** Signs and symptoms of mania (or a manic episode) include:

- Increased energy, activity, and restlessness

- An excessively "high," overly good, euphoric mood

- Extreme irritability, often aggressive, provocative, or intrusive behavior

- Reckless behavior, such as spending sprees, impulsive business decisions, erratic driving, and increased sex drive and sexual indiscretions

- Racing thoughts and talking very fast, jumping from one idea to another

- Distractibility, or lack of concentration

- The need for little sleep, as the person does not feel tired

- Unrealistic beliefs in one's abilities and powers (e.g., grandiose thoughts, inflated sense of self-importance)

- Poor judgment, impulsiveness with denial that anything is wrong

- Abuse of drugs, particularly cocaine, alcohol, and sleeping medications

## Making sense of manic patients

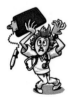

**Don't panic:** When we are faced with dealing with a manic patient who is out of control, it can easily make us feel out of control too. Here are a few things to keep in mind:

- The patient is being controlled by his or her disease. Control of behaviors and feelings is simply not possible.

- The patient lacks any insight into his or her behavior. People in manic states do not realize they are sick, and they are unaware of the consequences of their behavior. They reject any idea that any illness is involved, and they find excuses to try to make sense of what is going on around them.

- The patient with mania becomes frustrated, often with others who cannot keep up with him or her. The patient may lash out and show his or her frustration in inappropriate ways. It often appears that the patient knows exactly how to push your buttons, or knows the exact things about which you are most sensitive.

- The patient with mania is hyperalert. People in manic states are hypervigilant and are often aware of things going on in the environment that others do not pick up on.

## Ways to prevent cycling

When working with manic individuals, you need to help them prevent the exhaustive cycles they live through. Although that is not always possible, you can help them identify and attempt to avoid the triggers that may lead to a mood swing. One of the most important aspects of managing manic episodes is to stick to a routine.

You can also help patients:

- **Set realistic goals.** Having unrealistic goals can set up the individual for disappointment and frustration, which can trigger a manic episode. Advise the patient to do the best he or she can to manage his or her symptoms, but expect and be prepared for occasional setbacks.

- **Get help from family and/or friends.** Everyone needs help from family and/or friends during a manic episode, especially if he or she has trouble telling the difference between what is real and what is not real. Having a plan in place before any mood changes occur can help the individual's support network to make good decisions.

- **Make a healthy living schedule.** This is important for those with mood swings. Many people with manic episodes find that sticking to a daily schedule can help control their mood. Some examples include regular meal times, routine exercise or other physical activity, and practicing some sort of relaxation each night before bed. Also, you can help to provide a balanced diet for the patient, focusing on the basics: fruits, vegetables, and grains, and less fat and sugar. Exercise uses up some energy and helps a person sleep better. Help the patient develop an exercise plan that fits his or her lifestyle. While in the hospital, taking walks around the unit during the day may benefit the patient.

- **Get enough sleep.** Getting a good night's sleep may be a challenge for a person with mania. Being overtired or getting too much or too little sleep can trigger mania in many people. While the patient is under your care, make up a schedule for rest and relaxation before sleep. Have the patient go to sleep and get up at the same time every day, and relax by listening to soothing music, reading, or taking a bath. Do not allow the patient to watch TV in his or her room.

- **Reduce stress.** Anxiety can trigger mania in many people. Ask the patient what helps him or her relax. It might be calming music or a meditation tape. Avoid those things that hype people up, such as watching violent shows on TV or listening to loud music. Helping the person reduce stress in general at home and at work might help prevent episodes. Advise the patient to ask for help: A young mother may ask her spouse, family, or friend to take care of some of the housework. If the person's job is proving to be too much, he or she can scale back some responsibilities. Doing a good job is important, but avoiding a manic mood episode is more important.

- **Avoid stimulants, alcohol, and drugs.** Many people with mania may turn to substances to try to avoid a manic episode, or stimulating substances to elevate their mood. Up to 60% of people with mood disorders also have substance abuse problems. This self-medication may give them some temporary relief, but it will make their condition worse over time. Tell the patient to eliminate the use of caffeine, alcohol, and recreational drugs (Spearing).

- **Stick with treatment.** It's essential for people with mania to continue their medication and get regular checkups. It can be tempting to stop treatment because the symptoms go away. However, it is important to continue treatment as prescribed to avoid taking risks or having unpleasant consequences associated with a manic episode. If the patient has concerns about treatment or the side effects of medicines, talk with him or her and caution the patient not to adjust the medicines on his or her own.

## Jump the gun: Identifying triggers

Catching the mania in its beginning stages may prevent catastrophic occurrences. When admitting a patient with a history of mania, ask him or her to help you make a list of triggers and initial symptoms.

At first, mood swings may take you by surprise. But over time, patterns or signs of the beginning of a period of mania emerge.

**Listen up:** On one nursing unit, the staff noted that an adolescent male always started to talk about a cartoon character, the Tasmanian Devil, as the first sign of an impending manic episode. Being aware of the triggers can help you prepare for the episode.

 **Tip:** Aside from a shift in mood, here are some common triggers to look for in patients you expect might be heading toward mania:

- Waking up feeling refreshed after just a few hours of sleep

- Increased energy level

- Enhanced sex drive, as evidenced by sexual talk and flirting

- Elated self-esteem

- Reduced concentration with many thoughts

Sometimes certain situations trigger a manic episode, such as stressful times at work or during holidays. Also, look for seasonal patterns to a person's mood changes.

Monitor the patient's mood every day. Once you know the early warning signs, assess the patient's mood daily to see whether he or she may be heading for a mood swing. List the signs/symptoms on a flow sheet.

Advise the patient to keep a journal. Make note of big events, stresses, any changes in sleep or eating patterns, changes in medication dosage, and changes in energy levels.

 **Listen up:** Roberto, a male patient with mania, kept a journal over many months and plotted his nightly sleep patterns and mood. He saw a definite pattern in the quality and quantity of sleep and his mood, shared it with the healthcare team working with him, and was able to make a plan to prevent and work with the early stages of his manic episodes.

It is a good idea to involve family and friends in the care of those with mania. Having a plan to handle the beginning stages of an episode is vital for the family. (See the section "Strategy time: Develop a plan for relapse," in Chapter 9.)

## Nurses need help too

Caring for someone with mania can be enormously difficult and exhausting. The presence of a manic patient can wreck the entire nursing unit. Nursing staff members are often mania's forgotten victims. Mania can cause a boatload of emotions for the staff.

Helping someone with mania is a balancing act. On the one hand, you want to be supportive and sympathetic to the person, and on the other, you need to take care of yourself. There's no easy solution.

 **Tip:** Here are some tips that might help you cope when caring for someone with mania:

- **Learn as much as you can about the illness.** If you routinely work with manic patients, learn as much as you can by reading, talking with other health professionals, and talking with the patient and his or her family members about their experiences.

- **Listen.** Pay attention to what a patient has to say. Don't assume that you know what he or she is going through. Don't treat all emotions and feelings as though they are signs of an illness. The patient's point of view is valid.

- **Ask how you can help.** Sometimes things can be overwhelming to a person with mania. Reducing stress helps. Anticipating needs and offering help with activities of daily living may help as well.

- **Do things with the patient.** This helps reduce distractions and avoids confusion. Don't force the issue. Instead, use gentle persuasion as needed.

- **Express your own concerns.** However, don't blame the patient. Don't list all of his or her mistakes. Focus on how his or her actions make others feel and how they affect the situation.

- **Accept your limits.** Supporting the patient and family members is one thing. But remember that you can't tackle this single-handedly. Get other staff members involved. Take shifts. Ask for the help of the patient's family members or friends. Take breaks from the manic person.

- **Do not be critical.** Criticism can cause alienation and anger.

- **Do not make demands, threats, or ultimatums unless you are can follow through with them.** Set firm limits on behavior with consequences.

- **Remember to be supportive and loving.** For example, you might say things like "I know you are angry at me right now for disagreeing with you, but I'm trying to do what's best for you. I hope you trust me enough to accept my help." Or "You probably won't agree with this, but you are having a manic episode right now. I am telling you the truth about this."

- **Use the technique in *50 First Dates*.** In the movie *50 First Dates*, Lucy (played by Drew Barrymore) suffers from short-term memory loss. She has no memory from one day to the next. She needs to be reminded each day who she is and who the people are around her, so Dr. Henry Roth (played by Adam Sandler) makes a video to show Lucy her past, and leaves a note for her to play the tape each day upon awakening.

You can use the same technique with the manic patient who is symptom-free. Ask him or her to write on a card a description of what happens to him or her in the beginning stages of a manic episode, and what he or she needs to do to help him or herself. Here is a brief example:

"I am reading this card because I am having a manic episode. I keep it with me to help me during these times. The nurses are trying to help me stay focused. My job is to follow their requests."

# References

Jamison, K. (1993). *Touched with Fire: Manic-Depressive Illness and the Artistic Temperament.* New York: Free Press.

Spearing, M. (2002). "Bipolar Disorder." National Institute of Mental Health. Available at *www.nimh.nih.gov/publicat/bipolar.cfm*. Accessed June 2, 2007.

# Chapter 7

# Addictions come in all sizes

"Drug addiction is a brain disease that can be treated."—Nora D. Volkow, MD, Director, National Institute on Drug Abuse

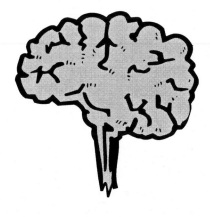

" . . . Addiction is a disease that affects both brain and behavior. We have identified many of the biological and environmental factors and are beginning to search for the genetic variations that contribute to the development and progression of the disease. . . . At the National Institute on Drug Abuse (NIDA), we believe that increased understanding of the basics of addiction will empower people to make informed choices in their own lives, adopt science-based policies and programs that reduce drug abuse and addiction in their communities, and support scientific research that improves the Nation's well-being" (Volkow).

## What is drug addiction?

**Drug addiction** is a chronic disease that is characterized by compulsive drug seeking and use, despite harmful consequences. The person with a drug addiction has periods of relapse and periods of recovery. Drug addiction changes the brain's structure and affects how it works. Brain changes from drug addiction last a long time, and can lead to the harmful behaviors and dangerous lifestyle seen in people who abuse drugs.

Addiction is similar to other diseases, such as heart disease. Both disrupt the normal, healthy functioning of the underlying organ, have serious harmful consequences, are preventable and treatable, and if left untreated, can last a lifetime (Volkow).

**Tip:** Why do people start to use drugs for recreation?

- To feel good or feel better

- To do better

- Out of curiosity

### Youths and recreational drugs

**Fact:** Teens and individuals with mental disorders are at greater risk of drug abuse, problem drinking, and other addictions than the general population (Volkow).

If you are a nurse who works with youth, log on to "The Cool Spot," a Web site made specifically for young teens to provide them with information about alcohol and help them handle peer pressure. Log on at *www.thecoolspot.gov*.

## Turning to alcohol

Although the overall prevalence of alcohol drinking decreased in the United States from 70% in 1984 to 65% in 1990, and heavy drinking—that is, consuming five or more drinks on one occasion at least weekly—also decreased from 6% to 4%, the prevalence of social problems as a result of drinking (problem drinking) has not shown a corresponding decline (10th special, National Institute on Alcohol Abuse and Alcoholism).

### What is problem drinking?

Not everyone who drinks alcohol regularly has a drinking problem, and not all problem drinkers drink every day. Problem drinkers:

- Feel irritable, resentful, or unreasonable when not drinking. And they often justify drinking as a way to calm themselves or to forget about their worries and concerns.

- Gulp drinks, and frequently have more than one drink a day. They gradually build up a tolerance, and they need to drink more alcohol to achieve the desired feeling.

- Lie about or try to hide their drinking habits.

- Hurt themselves, or someone else, while drinking.

- Have medical, social, or financial worries because of their drinking (National Institute on Aging).

A standard drink is generally considered to be 12 ounces of beer, 5 ounces of wine, or 1.5 ounces of 80-proof distilled spirits. Each of these drinks contains roughly the same amount of absolute alcohol—approximately 0.5 ounce or 12 grams (Moderate, National Institute on Alcohol Abuse and Alcoholism).

## Alcohol and the elderly

Many family members, friends, and nurses overlook problem drinking in older adults. Sometimes it is mistaken for other conditions, such as signs of dementia. You need to be alert for problem drinking in the elderly because the aging process affects how the body metabolizes alcohol: The same amount of alcohol can have a greater effect as a person grows older. In addition, certain health conditions, such as high blood pressure, ulcers, and diabetes, can worsen with alcohol use.

Using alcohol with medications can become dangerous for the older adult. Drinking alcohol while taking medications can cause harmful interactions, as well as forgetfulness and confusion. Here are some of the special precautions you can share with older adults:

- Aspirin and other medications can cause stomach ulcers and bleeding. The risk of bleeding is higher if the person takes aspirin.

- Many cold and allergy preparations cause drowsiness. The combination of these and alcohol may cause excessive drowsiness.

- Both alcohol and many over-the-counter (OTC) medications such as acetaminophen (Tylenol) are metabolized in the liver. As the number of medications a person takes increases, the chances of overtaxing the liver increase.

- Some OTCs, such as cough syrups, have a high alcohol content.

 **Fact:** The National Institute on Alcohol Abuse and Alcoholism, part of the National Institutes of Health, recommends that people over age 65 who choose to drink have no more than one drink per day. Drinking at this level usually is not associated with health risks.

## Beyond alcohol and drugs

A broad definition of addiction is that it is any activity, substance, object, or behavior that is the major focus of a person's life, excluding other activities, and causing harm to oneself or others. Addictions can be physical, such as a physical addiction to alcohol and nicotine. Addictions can also be psychological, such as an addition to gambling, sex, work, running, or shopping.

### Common characteristics of addictive behaviors

There are many common characteristics among the various addictive behaviors:

- **Obsession:** Constantly thinking of the object/activity/substance. With this comes a sense of loss of control over it. In addition, the person continues to engage in the activity in spite of causing harm.

- **Compulsion:** Doing it over and over. The person also may feel a sense of withdrawal when stopping.

- **Denial:** Denying the problem or the severity of the problem. Addicts give themselves good cover stories if they are found participating in the activity.

- **Harm:** Experiencing periods of memory loss (blackouts), as well as various physical problems. All addicts can suffer from various emotional disturbances, such as depression and low self-esteem.

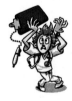 **Don't panic:** Why do some people become addicted?
Like other conditions, no single factor determines addiction. It is most likely a combination of biological makeup, surrounding environment, and genetic factors.

### Can addiction be treated successfully?

Yes, addiction can be treated successfully.

### Can addiction be cured?

Like other chronic diseases, addiction can be managed successfully, although not cured in the sense that the person need not ever deal with it again. Treatment of all chronic illnesses requires making lifestyle changes, and continued surveillance of the condition.

### Does relapse mean failure?

No, relapse does not mean failure. All chronic diseases have periods of relapse.

## Insight into intoxication

When working with an intoxicated person:

- First, assess the situation and make sure you know what you are dealing with.

- If the person is intoxicated on alcohol or drugs, get help. Intoxicated people are often unpredictable and may become violent without provocation.

- Provide for safety. Move the person to a safer environment and remove all harmful objects.

- Continually assess for signs of injury, such as head trauma, or the presence of other conditions such as hyperglycemia.

- Expect the unexpected. The intoxicated person may be very labile, crying one moment and charging the door in the next.

- Know the person's limitations. You cannot expect an intoxicated person to think rationally; therefore, do not try to reason with him or her, or trust his or her cooperation.

- Be patient. There is no need to escalate the situation by becoming loud and angry. Your calm presence may reassure the individual, who may be confused and frightened.

- Stay in control, professional, and emotionally detached.

- Set up the treatment that the person needs, including any supportive treatment while recovering from the intoxication.

## Answers for addicts

 Those with addictive behaviors, whether it is problem drinking, drug addiction, or another type of addiction, can be quite persuasive in their arguments. They might try to pin you down, often turning the conversation around to you rather than dealing with the addictive behavior. As a nurse, you need to avoid the common pitfalls.

Having pat answers to some of their statements can help. For example:

**"I need alcohol (cigarettes, drugs, to shop, etc.) to block my emotional pain."**

**Don't panic:** Say "Blocking emotional pain does not work. You are not alone. Everyone has emotional pain of some sort, and everyone needs to learn to deal with it."

**"I can't handle frustration and pain."**

**Don't panic:** Say "Handling frustration and pain can be learned. Developing a tolerance to frustration grows as you work with it."

**"I deserve to feel good and get high (have sex, gamble, smoke cigarettes, etc.)."**

**Don't panic:** Say "Everyone deserves to feel good, but not at the expense of their health or another's well-being."

**"I can't help it."**

**Don't panic:** Say "You are responsible for your behavior."

**"It is not my fault. I am an addict."**

**Don't panic:** Say "You are responsible for avoiding situations that cause you to relapse."

**"I'm no good; I am a failure."**

**Don't panic:** Say "You might feel that way now. I am not ready to accept that."

"I am in control of my drinking (gambling, running, etc.). I can stop anytime."

**Don't panic:** Say "What just happened now doesn't support that."

## The road to recovery

Sustaining hope is also an important ingredient when working with addicts. Chronic illnesses are, by definition, illnesses of remission and relapse. However, recall that any period without the addictive substance is a period of health.

- The longer the periods of remission, the more the body can heal

- The shorter the periods of relapse, the better for the body, as it reduces the amount of injury to it

So, as nurses, we need to keep perspective, and help our patients and their family members and loved ones do the same. A little hope and a bit of encouragement may bring the addict comfort and strength to continue in recovery.

## References

"10th Special Report to the U.S. Congress on Alcohol and Health." National Institute on Alcohol Abuse and Alcoholism. Available at *http://pubs.niaaa.nih.gov/publications/10report/intro.pdf*. Accessed June 3, 2007.

"AgePage: Alcohol Use and Abuse." National Institute on Aging. Available at *www.nia.nih.gov/HealthInformation/Publications/alcohol.htm*. Accessed June 3, 2007.

"Alcohol Alert: Moderate Drinking." National Institute on Alcohol Abuse and Alcoholism. Available at *http://pubs.niaaa.nih.gov/publications/aa16.htm*. Accessed June 3, 2007.

"Assessing Alcohol Problems." National Institute on Alcohol Abuse and Alcoholism. Available at *http://pubs.niaaa.nih.gov/publications/Assesing%20Alcohol/index.htm*. Accessed June 3, 2007.

Volkow, N. (2007). "Drugs, Brains, and Behavior—The Science of Addiction." National Institute on Drug Abuse. Available at *www.drugabuse.gov/scienceofaddiction/*. Accessed June 2, 2007.

# Part Two

Now that we've got a foundation to build on, it's time for some action. This section is chock full of hints, tips, techniques, and strategies to help you handle everything from anxiety and narcissism, to insomnia and suicide. Fill your nurse toolbox so you'll be ready in any situation.

# Chapter 8

# Laying the foundation for understanding behavior

Let's face it, most people go about their day doing one thing: trying to get their needs met. They try to meet their physical needs by providing themselves with shelter, food, and clothing; their emotional needs by searching out feelings of love and emotional comfort; and their spiritual needs by participating in activities that promote greater understanding of why things happen and determining the purpose of their lives. Theories of human behavior and growth and development have attempted to answer the question of why we do what we do, and how we go about our day getting our needs met. Let's quickly review some of the classic theories as a way to explain behavior.

## We are unaware (of most) of what we do

Sigmund Freud's concept of the conscious, preconscious, and unconscious mind, and how it resembles an iceberg, offers one example of how the mind works and influences behavior. The visible part of the iceberg is the **conscious mind**, what we are aware of at any particular moment: our present perceptions, memories, thoughts, fantasies, and feelings. Working closely with the conscious mind, and just below the surface, is the **preconscious mind**. It contains those things that are not in our awareness all of the time, but that can be brought into our awareness easily. The largest part of the iceberg and the part that is below the surface is the **unconscious mind** which contains all the things we are not aware of, including many things that Freud believed we can't bear to see, such as the memories and emotions associated with trauma. According to Freud, it is the unconscious part of us that drives our behavior (Freud, Boeree).

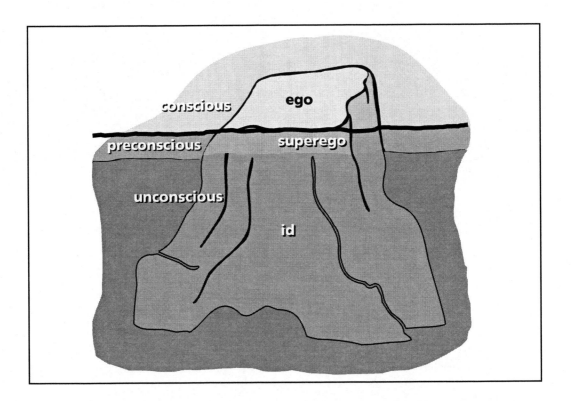

Freud also believed that the mind possessed three interacting thought systems: the id, the ego, and the superego. The **id** is sensitive to our needs (hunger, thirst, avoidance of pain, and desire for sex), and strives to keep us in a state of satisfaction or pleasure. In other words, it strives to keep us in a state where our needs are taken care of immediately, if not sooner. The hungry infant, screaming itself blue for food, is a good example of the id at work. An adult in pain may be another example of the id at work.

**Alarm:** Maureen, a nurse, had her daughter by cesarean section. She was told that the attending OB/GYN needed to give her the first doses of pain medication by IV push. She vividly recalls yelling out in a very direct voice: "I do not care what the attending is doing or where he is, I want him in here now to push that medication." Pure id at work.

In opposition to the id is the **superego**, which is sometimes called the internal parent. The superego is forever making judgments regarding what we have done right or wrong. It is the moral part of us that wants to "punish" us when we forget something, lose our cool at work, or don't perform "A" work.

A person's **ego** is the problem-solver. The ego understands that other people have needs and desires too, and that sometimes being impulsive or selfish, as the id wants to be, can hurt us in the long run. The ego tries to satisfy the id in appropriate ways, while keeping the superego in check, balancing its demands for perfection with the id's demands for immediate gratification.

Looking back at the illustration of the iceberg, both the id and the superego are underneath the surface of the water, meaning that their escapades are not within a person's awareness. So, in a nutshell, Freud tells us something most nurses are aware of: A lot of times the reason behind behavior is outside of our awareness. People cannot always say why they do what they do. No wonder things can get really messy at times!

## Reward me!

B. F. Skinner believed that a person's behavior was a result of past consequences of his or her behavior. Very simply, Skinner believed that people continue to do things for which they are rewarded, and stop doing things for which they are not rewarded.

Skinner also believed that individuals do things to avoid pain or punishment, which means that if a person is punished for a certain behavior, he or she will act in ways to avoid the punishment. An example is a nurse who learns not to be assertive with a certain supervisor because that supervisor responds negatively to assertive behavior. Instead, the nurse uses other ways to get his or her needs met. Sometimes these behaviors are adaptive, such as learning how to address concerns in an indirect way to the supervisor; or maladaptive, such as agreeing to something the supervisor requests, and then not doing it.

Skinner's theory basically boils down to praising or rewarding behaviors you want to see again, and ignoring or punishing behaviors you do not want to see again. Sound familiar? These are fairly basic concepts reviewed in many different situations from child rearing, patient teaching, and self-care management.

## Addressing our needs in order

Abraham Maslow placed an individual's needs in a hierarchy, believing that certain needs must be met before others. According to Maslow, needs at the base of the triangle must be satisfied before moving upward, with each step in the triangle needing to be met in succession. For example, a person cannot reach self-actualization, or becoming everything that he or she is capable of becoming, before getting all of his or her other needs met. Nurses know that you cannot teach a person a new procedure for self-care if the person is hungry, or sleepy, or in pain. Basic needs are taken care of before other, higher-level needs are attempted to be met.

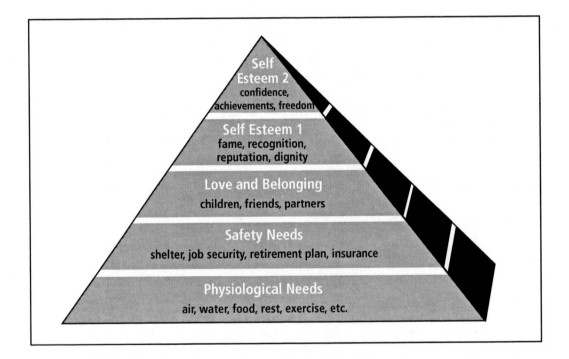

## Conflict equals development?

Erik Erickson described development in eight stages. In each stage, individuals grapple with a conflict, the outcome of which leads either to growth or to a negative outcome. Nurses, familiar with Erikson's stages, are well aware that people of all ages might still be working on unresolved issues of earlier stages of development, causing them to act in ways that interfere with their lives.

**Figure 1: Erickson's Stages of Development**

| Stages | Basic Development Task |
| --- | --- |
| **One:** The Infant: Trust vs. Distrust | Trust that basic needs will be met |
| **Two:** Toddlers: Autonomy vs. Shame and Doubt | Gain self-control and independence |
| **Three:** Childhood: Initiative vs. Guilt | Develop a sense of purpose and initiate one's own activities |
| **Four:** School Age: Industry vs. Inferiority | Achieve self-confidence |
| **Five:** Adolescence: Identity vs. Role Confusion | Develop a sense of self and self-mastery |
| **Six:** Young Adulthood: Intimacy vs. Isolation | Form lasting, loving relationships and commit to a cause |
| **Seven:** Adulthood: Generativity vs. Stagnation | Achieve life goals while thinking of future generations |
| **Eight:** Old Age: Ego Integrity vs. Despair | Review one's own life and feel good about one's self and accomplishments |

## Putting these theories to use

Using these theories in combination, nurses can come to understand human behaviors. By combining the concepts presented in these four theories, we can outline fairly accurately why people do what they do:

- We do what we do to get our needs met

- Our behavior is directed toward providing for our physical well-being, regaining emotional equilibrium, and answering questions of purpose

- Some, or most, of what we do is usually outside of our awareness

- We often respond to situations using behaviors that have worked for us in the past, and these learned behaviors may have become automatic responses for us; we use them even without thinking

- Some of what we deal with on a daily basis may have more to do with past experiences than with the present moment

- Taking care of basic needs is imperative, and focusing on higher-level needs occurs only after our most basic needs are met

- Life is a series of growth opportunities, the outcome of which leads to maturity and moving on

Theoretical understanding is a way of trying to comprehend something. Not being right or wrong—or good or bad—the concepts of the theory can be used by nurses to understand behavior and develop strategies to handle it in helpful and fulfilling ways. By recalling the basic concepts of human behavior, and observing it through the lenses of these concepts, you look at human behavior objectively and do not take what patients do as anything directed to you personally.

 **Tip:** Remember, a theory is not a fact. A theory is a way of trying to understand something. It is not right or wrong, or good or bad. A theory is made up of concepts, and they are usually reviewed separately so that we can understand them. However, no concept in a theory stands alone. Each is intertwined with the others. Likewise, no theory stands alone. Many different theories of growth and development as well as theories of personality, taken together, help explain why we do what we do.

## References

"Abraham H. Maslow: Books, Articles, Audio/Visual, & His Personal Papers." Abraham H. Maslow Publications. Available at *www.maslow.com*. Accessed June 3, 2007.

"A Brief Survey of Operant Behavior." B. F. Skinner Foundation. Available at *www.bfskinner.org/briefsurvey.html*. Accessed June 3, 2007.

Boeree, C. (2006). "Personality Theories: Erik Erikson." Available at *http://webspace.ship.edu/cgboer/erikson.html*. Accessed April 28, 2007.

Boeree, C. (2006). "Personality Theories: Sigmund Freud." Available at *http://webspace.ship.edu/cgboer/freud.html*. Accessed April 28, 2007.

Maslow, A. (1998). *Toward a Psychology of Being*, 3rd edition. New York: Wiley.

"The Freud Museum." Available at *www.freud.org.uk*. Accessed June 3, 2007.

# Chapter 9

# Working with people who are afraid or anxious

## The difference between fear and anxiety

Fear is usually defined as a natural response to a real danger. Everyone has experienced it at one time or another. The usual response to fear is to assess the situation, determine whether it is a real danger—as opposed to a misperception—and then take steps to handle the problem.

Fear may disrupt our lives. We may experience restless sleep, difficulty concentrating, or loss of appetite. However, most people are able to handle or avoid their fears and move on.

Here are some ways you can help patients handle their fears:

- Determine exactly what is causing the fear. Getting the patient's description of what he or she is afraid of is very important. Don't make assumptions.

- Caution the patient not to intensify the fear by his or her own self-talk.

- You can help the patient problem-solve his or her fear by asking the patient to answer the question "What is the worst that can happen?" Then, discuss with the patient whether he or she could live with that, or point out the odds of that happening.

- Ask the patient, "What is the most likely thing that can happen?" You can prompt the patient to visualize the situation and how he or she might respond, and offer alternatives as appropriate.

- Help the patient take actions that might protect him or her, if needed.

- Encourage the patient to decide for him or herself when he or she is ready to face the fear.

 **Listen up:** Cindy Keyser, a mother of five from Lancaster County, PA, puts it in perspective: "I say to my children, 'If you are afraid of getting water in your nose when jumping into the swimming pool, hold your nose.' It is as simple as that. When fears are recognized, they can often be overcome."

## The lowdown on disorders

But anxiety is another story. Constant anxiety can interfere with daily living and cause a wide variety of both physical and emotional illnesses. When anxiety is out of hand, it can become a serious medical illness. Serious forms of anxiety affect approximately 19 million American adults (Anxiety, NIMH).

Anxiety disorders are chronic and relentless, and can grow progressively worse if not treated. Here is a brief description of the most frequently occurring anxiety disorders:

- **Generalized anxiety disorder (GAD):** excessive, unrealistic worry that lasts for more than six months. Physical symptoms include trembling, insomnia, dizziness, and irritability.

- **Obsessive-compulsive disorder (OCD):** persistent, recurring thoughts that exaggerate anxiety or fears; the need to do something (compulsion) to rid oneself of the recurring thought (obsession). For more information about obsessive-compulsive behaviors, please see Chapter 13.

- **Panic disorder:** severe distress that causes the individual to believe he or she is having a health problem (such as a heart attack) or will lose control.

- **Post-traumatic stress disorder (PTSD):** a cluster of symptoms that persist after experiencing a traumatic event (war, sexual or physical assault, unexpected death of a loved one, disaster).

- **Social anxiety disorder:** an individual's extreme anxiety that he or she is being judged by others or a belief that he or she is behaving in a way that might cause embarrassment (Anxiety, NIMH).

## The role of the brain

The amygdala and the hippocampus play significant roles in the production of both fear and anxiety:

- The **amygdala** is an almond-shaped structure deep in the brain that is believed to be a communication hub between the parts of the brain that process incoming sensory signals and the parts that interpret these signals. Emotional memories are believed to be stored in the amygdala and these may play a role in anxiety disorders involving very distinct objects or activities, such as dogs, spiders, or flying.

- The **hippocampus** is the part of the brain that encodes threatening events into memories. The hippocampus has been shown to be smaller in some people who were victims of child abuse or who served in the military. Further research is needed to determine what role the hippocampus plays in flashbacks, memory deficits, and fragmented memories of the traumatic events that are common in people with some anxiety disorders, such as PTSD (Anxiety, NIMH).

In general, anxiety disorders are treated with medication, specific types of psychotherapy, or both. The principal medications used for anxiety disorders are antidepressants and antianxiety medications. Beta blockers, such as propranolol (Inderal) and atenolol (Tenormin), are also used in severe anxiety disorders to help control physical symptoms, such as palpitations.

## The importance of being anxious

It is a slight motivational type of anxiety that gets us out and going everyday. It is a mild anxiety that prompts us to our top performance. Some people believe that if we had no anxiety, we might just lie around all day doing nothing. Mild forms of anxiety are not perceptible to others. Speech teachers often tell students: "It's okay that your knees shake behind the podium when you are giving your speech. No one can see it and only you know it is happening."

You can do the best for your patient by assessing his or her level of anxiety and providing the appropriate interventions.

## Assessing level of anxiety and interventions

This table can help you determine your patient's level of anxiety and what you can do to relieve it.

### Figure 2: Assessing levels of anxiety

| Level of Anxiety | Physical Symptoms | Cognitive/Perceptual Manifestations | Interventions |
|---|---|---|---|
| **Mild** | Some muscle tension. | ↑ alertness. ↑ awareness. Peak performance. | Help talk out situation as needed. Listen. |
| **Moderate** | Moderate muscle tension. ↑ BP, P, R. Feeling nervous and jittery. | ↓ ability to communicate. Misperceptions. Confusion. | All of the above, as needed. Offer simple choices. Give clear directions. Offer physical outlet. Breathe into a paper bag. |
| **Severe** | Extreme muscle tension. Physical symptoms (heart pounding, sweating, etc.) may cause more alarm. | Distorted perceptions. Disoriented. | All of the above, as needed. Orient to surroundings. Correct any misperceptions. Medications may be needed. |
| **Panic** | Muscle tension increases to the point of needing to move, often aimlessly, sometimes violently. | Overwhelmed. Terrified. | All of the above, as needed. Safety is first concern. Call for help. Medication is usually required. |

### A word about paranoia

**Paranoia**, or paranoid delusions, are the presence of extreme fears, usually associated with a disorder of thought, such as drug-induced paranoia or the diagnosis of paranoid schizophrenia, or panic disorder. The person's fears can come from misinterpretations of what is going on around him or her, the presence of auditory or visual hallucinations, or extreme anxiety. However, it is important to note that not all fears expressed by a person with a mental illness are a product of paranoid delusions. Sometimes there is some basis for the person's fear. Many people with schizophrenia and other mental disorders that interfere with a person's ability to think clearly have been victims of violence and ridicule and/or have been taken advantage of by others in some way. It is important for you to check out what the person tells you is bothering him or her. Verify what you have been told with others, and ask other staff members to talk with the patient to reach a consensus about the patient's level of concern.

## Strategy time: Develop a plan for relapse

People with chronic illnesses may experience additional anxiety during periods of relapse of their illness because of concerns about their family and/or their own welfare. Helping them develop a plan to follow during relapse may alleviate some of their anxiety. When their symptoms are well controlled, work with them to develop a treatment plan to share with their family members and healthcare providers when they begin to show signs of relapse. Then, when they need to rely on others for help, they will be assured that they still have some say in the plan of their care.

A plan of action includes specific items that need to be addressed during relapse. It is important to consider all of the patient's daily responsibilities when developing the plan of action, and it may take some time to address all concerns. Include these in the plan:

- The patient's wishes for the care of children, pets, and plants, if needed

- Who the patient wants to manage his or her business, pay bills, and handle financial matters

- What treatment facility and care providers the person would like to attend to him or her

- Who needs to be notified, and how best to contact them

Plans of action can also include the following documents:

- An advance directive for treatment, which is written during remission to help outline treatment during relapse. An advance directive can be very useful, particularly when symptoms of fear, suspicion of others, or paranoia emerge in those with mental disorders.

- A durable power of attorney, which designates who will be in charge of making decisions when the patient cannot make decisions for him or herself.

- A power of attorney for managing financial records when the patient is unable to do so. He or she may want someone to cosign important items such as home mortgages (WebMD).

## References

"Anxiety Disorders." National Institute of Mental Health. Available at *www.nimh.nih.gov/publicat/anxiety.cfm*. Accessed June 2, 2007.

"Develop a Plan for Relapse of Schizophrenia." WebMD. Available at *www.webmd.com/hw-popup/Develop-a-plan-for-relapse-of-schizophrenia*. Accessed June 2, 2007.

Ho, B. C., et al. (2003). "Schizophrenia and other psychotic disorders." *Textbook of Clinical Psychiatry*, 4th edition. Washington, DC: American Psychiatric Publishing.

# Chapter 10

# Pay attention to this chapter: Dealing with ADHD

Attention-deficit/hyperactivity disorder (ADHD) is usually seen in preschool children and those in their early school years. It is estimated that 3–5%, or approximately 2 million children in the United States, have ADHD (NIMH). However, ADHD is not a disorder that affects only children. Several studies done in recent years estimate that 30–70% of children with ADHD continue to exhibit symptoms in the adult years (Silver).

ADHD has three cardinal characteristics: inattention, hyperactivity, and impulsivity. Let's take a closer look:

- Children who are inattentive have a hard time keeping their minds on any one thing and may get bored quickly. They are easily distracted, make careless mistakes, and have problems following instructions carefully and completely. They may go from one uncompleted task to another.

- Hyperactive children always seem to be in constant motion. They squirm and fidget. Hyperactive teenagers or adults may feel internally restless, and may feel as though they need to stay busy.

- Impulsive children often blurt out inappropriate comments, and have a hard time waiting for things they want. Teens and adults may do things that have an immediate payoff rather than stick with activities that take more time and effort but, in the end, provide greater benefit to them.

There are numerous theories about what causes ADHD, including the use of cigarettes and alcohol during pregnancy. High levels of lead may also increase the risk of ADHD. (Thus, the regulations against the use of lead-based paint.) The connection between ADHD and ingesting sugar or food additives, however, has not been proven.

Genetics can also play a role, as ADHD often runs in families. Now, studies on the disorder focus on brain structure and function. In research conducted at the National Institute of Mental Health (NIMH), children with ADHD showed about 4% smaller brain volumes in their frontal lobes, temporal gray matter, caudate nucleus, and cerebellum.

## Try these treatments

Treatments for ADHD include medication management and behavioral treatment. Structuring a patient's environment and being consistent in your approach can be helpful. Here are some hints to use when working with children with ADHD:

- Provide a schedule and routine in their day. Post the schedule where it can be readily seen.

- Organize their belongings. Have a place for everything and keep everything in its place.

- Write down important items that you want them to remember.

- Provide consistent rules that they can understand and follow. When rules are followed, give rewards, like praise, hugs, or high fives.

- Be the child's advocate. Helping others understand the reason for the child's behavior protects his or her self-esteem.

Teens with ADHD can present you with additional challenges. As the nurse, it is important for you to make sure the teen understands the rules for his or her behavior. Rules need to be straightforward and easy to understand. Posting rules along with the schedule for the day is helpful. If rules are broken, or the teen does not perform as expected in his or her care, present the discrepancy in a calm, matter-of-fact manner.

When working with adults with ADHD, either as patients or as colleagues, here are a few things that will help:

- Reduce distractions when talking with them, or give them assignments or directions.

- Clearly define what is expected of them.

- Give them time to learn and practice any tasks or skills expected of them.

- Present instructions verbally as well as in writing. Provide handouts and visual aids. Break information down into small steps.

- Allow them to take notes or tape-record important information.

- Give them the opportunity to ask questions and state back important information.

 **Tip:** Check out these books for more information on ADHD:

- *Taking Charge of ADHD*, by Russell A. Barkley, PhD

- *ADHD: Attention-Deficit Hyperactivity Disorder in Children and Adults*, by Paul H. Wender, MD

- *Straight Talk about Psychiatric Medications for Kids*, by Timothy E. Wilens, MD

## References

"Attention Deficit Hyperactivity Disorders." National Institute of Mental Health. Available at *www.nimh.nih.gov/publicat/adhd.cfm*. Accessed July 29, 2007.

Bruyère, S. M. (Ed.) (2001). "Working Effectively with People with Attention Deficit/ Hyperactivity Disorder." Ithaca, NY: Cornell University. Available at *http://digitalcommons.ilr.cornell.edu/edicollect/19*. Accessed July 30, 2007.

Silver, L. (2000). "Attention-deficit hyperactivity disorder in adult life." *Child and Adolescent Psychiatric Clinics of North America*, 9(3): 411–523.

# Chapter 11

# Delving into defense mechanisms

Using Freudian concepts to understand human behavior, one could say that the ego often has a hard time pleasing the id and keeping the superego in check. So, it has developed a way to reduce anxiety through the use of ego defense mechanisms, those things that unconsciously block or distort our thoughts and beliefs into more acceptable, less threatening ones.

Ego defense mechanisms (sometimes called coping or protective mechanisms) are, in short, used to protect the ego from full awareness of the situation. Their purpose is to help the person cope with a situation that he or she might not be able to handle.

Using defense mechanisms is a common human trait. We all use them. Some defense mechanisms are considered to be more helpful than others. Others may cause more problems for the person using them, in terms of creating unhealthy or unfulfilled relationships or losing touch with reality.

Most nurses are very familiar with defense mechanisms, having learned them early in their nursing school careers. Let's review some of the most common ego defense mechanisms and see how they apply to patient situations.

## Figure 3: Examples of defense mechanisms

| Defense Mechanism | Definition | Example |
|---|---|---|
| Denial | Protecting self from reality | Thinking the high cholesterol level was a lab error. |
| Fantasy | Imaginary achievements | Describing impossible situations: "My baby was walking at three months." |
| Repression | Preventing painful memories/thoughts from entering consciousness | Forgetting what he or she was told about a chronic illness. |
| Rationalization | Giving a good cover story, justifying what one did | Saying something like "I don't come to every appointment late." |
| Projection | Pointing the finger at others instead of ourselves | Saying something like "You always try to con me into getting what you want." |
| Reaction formation | Adopting opposing attitudes and beliefs | Agreeing to do what is asked when the opposite is true. |
| Displacement | Taking things out on others | Yelling at a child after being given a bad diagnosis. |
| Insulation | Withdrawing emotionally | Not responding emotionally to a child's injury. |
| Intellectualization | Using logic and rational thought when expression of feelings is too painful | Saying something like "Research does not support that." |
| Undoing | Atoning for something done | Bringing the nurses candy after having an anger episode in the nurses' station. |
| Regression | Returning to an earlier stage of development | Crying and refusing to discuss discharge planning. |
| Identification | Taking on attributes of others | Acting like a staff member as a way to deal with feelings of inferiority. |
| Compensation | Covering up weaknesses by emphasizing other traits | Telling the nurse all he or she knows about a certain condition rather than admitting that he or she cannot read the information given about the disorder. |

Rational problem-solving is not a defense mechanism. Oftentimes, rational problem-solving is enough to resolve an issue. Then, the use of defense mechanisms is not needed.

**Tip:** A well-rounded person, a mature individual, usually has little need to use ineffective or maladaptive ego defense mechanisms. However, when people are sick, have just been given bad news, have a loved one injured, or are uncomfortable for whatever reason, even the most sophisticated resort to the use of defense mechanisms to help them get through.

## Find some common ground

How do you relate to a person who is using a defense mechanism?

- Recognize that the use of defense mechanisms is to protect the mind from total awareness of the gravity of the situation.

- Avoid hurrying someone along, as this only creates more frustration and confusion. Sometimes the person is able to develop awareness little by little.

- Provide a safe environment for the patient so that he or she might feel more comfortable doing the emotional work that is needed given the situation.

- Be aware of how you are reacting and try to maintain a professional stance. Don't get hooked into the patient's mini-drama.

- Provide information that might help clarify the situation.

- Stop giving information when you see that it frustrates or overwhelms the patient.

- Maintain a quiet voice and comforting physical appearance.

- Give the person some emotional space as well as the physical space needed to soothe him or her.

- Provide for the patient's basic needs.

- Say things like "I am available if you want to talk about this more later."

- Work around the use of the defense mechanism if possible.

- Avoid the tendency to take the use of defense mechanisms by others personally.

- Be patient and wait to see whether the person is able to address the issue in a more mature fashion later.

## Let's chat about personality traits

Personality traits are what make each person unique. For example, some people have bubbly personalities, whereas others are more laid-back. Most of us can identify personality traits in others more readily than we can in ourselves. Usually a person can adjust his or her dominant personality traits to fit the occasion. For example, a bubbly person could act more serious in a serious situation.

However, some people's traits are more fixed and rigid, and they cannot adjust them as needed. When a person has such deeply rooted personality traits that they become inflexible and the person cannot adjust his or her approach when it is needed, this is called a **personality disorder**.

People with fixed personality traits often have difficulty in interpersonal relationships, including their work situation. And people with fixed personality traits are the most challenging for counselors and others working with them. Fixed personality traits are an integral part of what defines them and influences their self-perceptions. Counseling most often focuses on reducing their anxiety, and increasing their coping and interpersonal skills.

In general, most people try to put forward their best behavior. When anxiety goes up, people may have a hard time controlling their behaviors. Each one of us has a certain way we typically behave when anxious. Some of us cry, some of us get quiet, and some of us may use defense mechanisms of projection or denial. Those with fixed personality traits become more fixed in their traits, even if doing so hinders them rather than helps them. So, the greater the anxiety, the more fixed and rigid the person becomes. What do you think is the way to handle people with rigid personality traits? Yes, you're right: It is to reduce their anxiety. They can relax a bit, and so can you.

 **Tip:** In general, when working with people with fixed personality traits, you can focus on reducing their overall anxiety by anticipating their needs, offering explanations for all you do with and/or to them, and answering any questions they pose.

You can also use the techniques you learned in Chapter 9 regarding how to work with people who are afraid and anxious. However, note that in some instances, you might need to do a bit more than that. The following chapters will look at ways to approach people who have some of the most common fixed personality traits.

## References

Boeree, C. (2006). "Personality Theories: Sigmund Freud." Available at *http://webspace.ship.edu/cgboer/freud.html*. Accessed April 28, 2007.

Freud, A. (1983). *The Ego and the Mechanisms of Defense: The Writings of Anna Freud, Vol. 1*. New York: International Universities Press.

"The Freud Museum." Available at *www.freud.org.uk*. Accessed June 3, 2007.

# Chapter 12

# Personality types that wreak havoc

T. S. Eliot aptly described some people as not wishing to do harm, but causing harm nonetheless as they are so "absorbed in the endless struggle to think well of themselves." Such a description could define those who are narcissistic. For them, life's events are always centered on them; and all that occurs is "all about me."

## Narcissism: It's all about me

People who are narcissistic:

- Have a sense of self-importance as evidenced by exaggerating their achievements

- Believe that only certain people are able to understand them

- Require excessive positive attention and special treatment

- Have a preoccupation with fantasies about their achievements and positive attributes

- Exploit others, show arrogance, and exhibit naughty attitudes and behaviors

- Lack empathy for others and can be envious of others, or believe others envy them

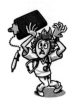

### Dealing with narcissistic behavior

**Don't panic:** Here are some ways to cope with narcissistic behavior in your patients:

- When explaining something, point out how it will benefit them.

- Recognize that their perception of you will be clouded by their self-centeredness.

- Be firm, but kind. Stay focused on their care, and do not stray into casual conversation.

- Listen quietly to what they have to say. There is no need to agree. Just listen.

- Take frequent breaks from them and ask others for help as needed.

- Don't take their comments to heart.

- Recognize that their inflations of themselves are most likely a way to cover up their feelings of inadequacies.

- Be professional and straightforward.

## Histrionics: Throwing a fit

A histrionic (or sometimes called hysterical) personality has a pattern of excessive emotionality and attention-seeking behavior.

Like Albert Goldman (played by Nathan Lane) in *The Birdcage*, a histrionic person can exhibit excessive behaviors. For example, Goldman bursts into tears, swishes his clothes as he moves, overdrinks, overexaggerates, and walks with a very prominent flair.

**Tip:** A mnemonic you can use to remember the criteria for histrionic personality is **PRAISE ME**:

> **P:** Provocative (or seductive) behavior
> **R:** Relationships, considered more intimate than they are
> **A:** Attention, must be at center of
> **I:** Influenced easily
> **S:** Speech (style), wants to impress, lacks detail
> **E:** Emotional liability, shallowness
>
> **M:** Makeup, physical appearance used to draw attention to self
> **E:** Exaggerated emotions, theatrical (Pinkofsky)

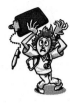

### Handling histrionic behavior

**Don't panic:** Here are some hints on how to handle histrionic behavior in your patients:

- Don't give them an audience, because they like to draw attention to themselves.

- Recognize that their affections are shallow and don't take offense if they tell every nurse they are the best nurse on the unit.

- Remember that they may exaggerate their symptoms, and their reactions to medications and treatments. As a nurse, you need to do a thorough assessment and avoid discounting their concerns.

- Although they may be able to develop rapport easily, you might recognize that they may come across as fake or shallow. They may be unable to display a wide range of depth of emotion.

- Be supportive, but resist the urge to rescue them. This may occur as they may seek constant reassurance and express the need to be rescued from their day-to-day problems, which they might express in very dramatic terms.

- Set clear boundaries, especially with people of the opposite sex, as they may become sexually provocative.

- Set clear expectations of their behavior and the limits of your involvement with them.

## Borderline personality: Stirring up the pot

**Fact:** Borderline personality disorder affects approximately 2% of the general population. About 75% of those diagnosed with borderline personality disorder are females (American Psychiatric Association).

You know you have a borderline personality on your unit if the nursing staff is in conflict over the patient's care. Some staff members want to rescue the patient, feel sorry for him or her, and overcare for the patient, whereas other staff members want to put the patient in his or her place, lay down the law, and avoid the patient. If the staff spends a lot of time talking about a particular patient, chances are the patient has a borderline personality.

A person with a borderline personality has very unstable relationships. This pattern is present throughout the person's life—it is repeated at work, at home, and in social situations. The person's emotions fluctuate back and forth quickly, and it is hard to keep up with him or her.

The person may come across as shallow, impulsive, and judgmental. For a person with a borderline personality, there is no gray, only black and white. You are either a friend or a foe.

People with a borderline personality make frequent suicidal gestures, express frequent suicidal thoughts, and can participate in self-mutilating behavior.

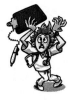

## Being comfortable with borderline patients

**Don't panic:** Here are some ways that you can reduce the amount of havoc borderline patients can cause on a nursing unit:

- Because they often are not able to distinguish between reality from their own misperceptions of the world and their surrounding environment due to their overwhelming emotions, it is important to be clear in all communications with them.

- Because they often see others in black-and-white terms, they are prone to split the staff into two opposing teams: those who want to rescue the patient and those who want to set limits on him or her. Thus, it is most important that the entire team gets together behind closed doors, not with the patient, to write a treatment plan that everyone agrees to follow.

- Be on guard so as to not get sucked into a staff-splitting struggle. You need to be steadfast in following the treatment plan and not allow yourself to be seduced by the patient's behaviors and pleas.

- Because they have a strong fear of being abandoned by others, borderline patients tend to cling to others. But because they also have poor interpersonal skills, they often push people away rather than draw them near. Be aware of their fear of abandonment, and set times when you will return to care for them. Then, make sure you are on time.

- Recognize that they may display extreme and confusing behaviors of both overpossessiveness of certain staff, and then being unavailable.

- Be aware that these patients are good at bringing out many negative feelings in others. Get support from the other staff members, ask for guidance from your supervisor, or request a consult from the mental health staff on how to better handle the situation with this patient.

- Assessing for suicide is important. If suicidal thoughts are expressed, institute the safety measures laid out in Chapter 17.

# References

"Narcissism 101." Available at *www.narcissism101.com*. Accessed June 3, 2007.

"Personality disorders." *Diagnostic and Statistical Manual of Mental Disorders*, 4th edition. Washington, DC: American Psychiatric Association.

"Personality Disorders." MentalHelp.net. Available at *www.mentalhelp.net/poc/ center_index.php?id=8&cn=8*. Accessed June 3, 2007.

Pinkofsky, H. B. (1997). "Mnemonics for DSM-IV personality disorders." *Psychiatry Services*, Sept., 48(9):1197–1198.

# Chapter 13

# Behaviors that drive you bananas

Does a certain group of patients simply drive you bananas? Sometimes you can't put your finger on it. Something just doesn't fit for you. Then, someone points it out to you by saying, "Don't you see how he or she is manipulating you?" Oh, that's it! He or she is a manipulator and the problem is solved. Or is it? What is manipulation? How does it get in the way? Can it ever be a good thing?

## Persuasion, influence, and manipulation: What's the difference?

Persuasion and influence are often seen as positive traits. We look at people who seem to be able to encourage others to get things done and wish we could be more like them. Indeed, very popular books have been written that teach others how to persuade or influence others. For example, there is a famous book by Dr. Jerome Frank—now updated by his daughter Julia—called *Persuasion and Healing*. It elucidates the positive influence of therapeutic relationships and other psychological healing techniques. In addition to this classic for healthcare providers, numerous pop books on the market give lots of hints on how to stop arguments by persuasion, get projects completed by influence and persuasion, and further your career by using your influence and persuasion.

### More about manipulation

Look back to Chapter 8, where we discussed why people do what they do. That chapter contained a list of the basic concepts of human behavior, which included the following:

- We do what we do to get our needs met

- Our behavior is directed toward providing for our physical well-being, regaining emotional equilibrium, and answering questions of purpose

- Some, or most, of what we do is usually outside of our awareness

- We often respond to situations using behaviors that have worked for us in the past, and these learned behaviors may have become automatic responses for us—we use them even without thinking

- Some of what we deal with on a daily basis may have more to do with past experiences than with the present moment

So, whether we call it persuasion, influence, or manipulation, people do what they do in order to get their needs met. And in providing for their well-being, they are often unaware of their own behavior. If it worked for them in the past, they do it again.

Now, there is a danger in using learned behaviors to get our needs met. Maybe some of these behaviors worked well for us as children but don't work so well as adults. Maybe some of the behaviors we learned were not very healthy behaviors.

When these behaviors become fixed—meaning that the person uses them all the time, in every situation (even in situations in which they are considered inappropriate)—that's when they get in the way and disturb others. They become maladaptive rather than adaptive. They lead to not getting one's needs met, chaotic interpersonal relationships, and unpleasant mini-dramas for all those concerned.

## Bothersome behaviors

Rather than using the label "manipulation," let's refine the definition and talk about the specific behaviors that drive us bananas. Then, let's look at ways to handle these behaviors in our work situations.

Whether we see them in patients or our peers, the following are some behaviors that cause distress in the workplace.

**Alarm:** First, we have the overt types of behavior that come across as verbal violence. These are often easier to handle because they are so overt. It is hard to miss them. They include:

- Making demands: "I must have this weekend off to attend my cousin's graduation," or "I can't go to x-ray until after I have my shower and shave."

- Violating rules and routines: A staff member consistently comes back from break or lunch late. A patient's family member brings in food from home, even after being told that the patient is presently on a very restricted diet.

- Making threats: "I'll throw this food tray at you if you come any closer."

Then, we have the more passive types of behavior that are meant to persuade you to do what the person wants. These might be harder to spot. If you grew up with adults who used these, you may even think they are healthy behaviors. Once pointed out to you, however, they may become more obvious.

**Alarm:** Here are a few behaviors that can drive you bananas but are harder to recognize at first:

- Eliciting pity: The staff member who says, "You just don't understand how hard it is for me to take care of that patient . . . ," but says this often about all kinds of patients. Or the person who is abusing drugs: "If you had my horrible upbringing you would take drugs to numb your pain, too. Can't you see how tough my life has been?"

- Ingratiating and flattering: The person who is always commenting on your clothes, your jewelry, and how good you look. Or the patient who says, "You are the best nurse on this floor. I don't know what I would do if you took a day off."

- Evoking guilt feelings: When people say, "If you had called me over the weekend like you said you were going to, this would never have happened," or "If you had made your rounds earlier like you usually do, I wouldn't be in this mess."

- Abusing compassion: When patients say, "You acted like you were a caring person and said that you would have a hard time on a restricted diet, so why are you making such a fuss over my wife bringing me food from home?"

- Attempting to exchange roles: When someone says, "I see that you have a problem with your weight. I am a fitness trainer and can help you with a personal plan to get you in shape. When you get a chance, come back and we'll start on it."

- Pitting people against each other: When a peer says, "That night shift is something else. I don't see them making rounds or doing any of the things I know they should be doing at night. You guys and gals on the day shift are top-notch." Or when a patient says, "Who is that young doctor who came in here yesterday anyway? I bet you know a heck of a lot more about my condition than he does."

- Questioning competence or authority: When a patient says, "Now, honey, you just go take care of your other patients, and send in the charge nurse. I need a real nurse in here to answer my questions."

- Being overly dependent: People who allow others to do for them, do not accept self-responsibility, and then skirt responsibility if things go wrong. They say things such as "I am sure you know best. Just take care of that for me. I rely on all you nurses to make sure I get better."

- Using avoidance: People who change the subject when it comes up, avoid being around people they dislike, or are silent rather than open with their opinions. When they do speak, it is in order to avoid: "I can't be on the same team as Susan. We don't work well together."

## Outlining obsessions and compulsions

It's also important to pay some attention to obsessive-compulsive behaviors. More specifically:

- **Obsessions** are thoughts that occur over and over again

- **Compulsions** are acts the person performs as a way to deal with the obsessive thoughts

Obsessive-compulsive behaviors are most often seen in one of the anxiety disorders, called obsessive-compulsive disorder (OCD). The etiology behind these behaviors is different from what we have been talking about. Anxiety is its root. People with OCD develop rituals that need to be completed in a certain way each time.

**Listen up:** Courtney, a nursing student, once took care of a woman who had a very elaborate ritual whenever she went to the bathroom: It consisted of the usual hand washing, but also included an inspection of her underwear for any contamination, washing her perineum with soap and water, and using powder to avoid the chance of an odor. Now, Courtney would have been okay handling this, but the patient had urinary frequency, and it seemed like she and the patient were in the bathroom most of the day. When Courtney tried to intervene or shorten the ritual, the patient became even more anxious. The only way to handle this situation was to work through it with patience. Courtney's nursing instructor reminded her that the ritual was a coping mechanism for dealing with extreme anxiety, and as the patient became more comfortable in her new surroundings and the medication to treat her urinary urgency took effect, the bathroom rituals would become less frequent. In the meantime, Courtney concentrated on making sure that the patient was as comfortable as possible, answering all her questions, and including her in all aspects of her care.

Common rituals include checking things, touching things, or counting things. An example of a common obsession is having a thought that you might have run over someone on a dark street at night, and then retracing the car route to make sure. You can see how this can get out of hand, because each time you go back to check, you may have run over someone again.

Anyone can have rituals. For example, I need to check all the drawers and under the bed "one last time" before I leave a hotel room. The difference is that the rituals performed by people with OCD greatly interfere with their lives. Many adults with OCD know the rituals are senseless.

## Hints for caring for people with OCD
When caring for people with OCD:

- Work under the premise that anything that increases anxiety will increase the likelihood of needing to participate in the rituals. See Chapter 9 for ways to handle anxiety.

- Displaying anger or frustration does not help.

- Ask the person to tell you how he or she has been taught to handle the rituals.

- Give the person plenty of time to get ready for procedures and daily activities.

## References

"Anxiety Disorders." National Institute of Mental Health. Available at
*www.nimh.nih.gov/publicat/anxiety.cfm*. Accessed June 10, 2007.

Fosset, B., M. Nadler-Moodie, and M. Thobaben (2004). *Psychiatric
Principles and Applications for General Patient Care*, 4th edition.
Brockton, MA: Western Schools.

Frank, J. D., and J. B. Frank (1993). *Persuasion and Healing: A Comparative
Study of Psychotherapy*, 3rd edition. Baltimore: The Johns Hopkins
University Press.

# Chapter 14

# Hints for working with ANY problem behavior

No matter the type of behavior, there are some general hints that can help you:

- **First, recognize the problem behavior.** If you have been making excuses for the person or the behavior, stop doing this. Use your nursing assessment skills to list the objective data you have about the behavior and the situation.

- **Organize the staff and plan for a consistent approach.** Talk with others you are working with and ask whether they have noticed the same behavior. If not, ask them to spend some time with the person, to make their own assessment. Point out the objective behaviors you have identified. Then, have a care-planning session (it need not be long) to decide how to approach the problem. Get help from more experienced nurses or from your supervisor as needed. Request an interdisciplinary team meeting if the issues of concern cross over into other departments working on your floor, such as dietary or the primary care provider. A plan that combines the following concepts works best:

  – Set clear limits on the behavior. Make sure the patient knows what is expected of him or her. Write out expectations if needed. Negotiate if there is room for negotiating. List responsibilities for all included.

– Be firm but kind. Try saying things like "We have some rules on the unit that all patients need to abide by. Not abiding by the rules causes confusion."

– Set the natural consequences for the behavior. Say something like "Not being on time for your appointment will probably result in you not being able to be seen. You will need to reschedule your appointment." Or "Not giving the specimen is your choice. However, by not giving it, we may not be able to diagnose you correctly."

– Ask the patient to accept personal responsibility. Say something like "Continuing to smoke in the bathroom jeopardizes the safety of you and everyone else on the unit. If you smoke again, the team has determined that our only recourse is to discharge you."

- **Refuse to allow staff members to deviate from the plan.** When dealing with disruptive behaviors on the unit, it is imperative that every team member follows the plan. If someone says he or she disagrees, ask whether he or she can agree to try the plan. Even if this person disagrees with it, ask him or her to try it for a few days to help the team and see whether it works.

- **Don't get sucked into the person's mini-drama.** Let's say you have recognized a problem with a patient's behavior. Others tell you that they noticed that behavior too, but that it is not a problem for them. This might be something that you need to work through. Others with more experience may not be so easily swayed by the behavior. Ask for guidance from other, more experienced nurses, or your supervisor. Don't be reluctant to try new behaviors. Test out others' suggestions and see how they fit. If needed, ask the other person to role-model the approach you want to try with the patient for you.

- **Differentiate the behavior from the patient.** Always remember to separate the behavior from the patient. It is the behavior that is ineffective and maladaptive. Calling the patient names or generalizing that he or she is a "bad" person does not help you handle the behavior. Writing off the patient does not help you, the patient, or anyone else.

- **Avoid arguing with the person.** The first step in avoiding an argument is to listen to the patient's concerns. Listen to understand; don't listen to reply. Once you think you understand, repeat the concerns back to the patient to make sure you got them right. Say something like "Let me see if I got it straight. You are upset about not having your tray on time.

You worry that if it is not on time you will have problems with your blood sugar. And you wonder why the staff members on the unit don't see the significance of you not getting your tray on time." Simply stating back what you heard and asking the patient to follow you is one way to reduce his or her anxiety and defuse the interaction.

**Watch out:** Some patients just want to argue. They are argumentative about everything. Simply say something like "I am not much on arguing. If you continue to argue, I will need to leave the room. But of course, if I leave I will not be able to help you. What can we do about this problem?"

- **Positively reinforce positive behaviors.** Even people with behaviors that disturb you have positive traits. Point out to the person times when you see him or her doing what is expected. Say something like "I see you are ready on time for your physical therapy appointment today. Thanks. It really helps keep things moving along on the unit."

**Tip:** At a lecture, a spiritual advisor answered a young man who asked how a person could start to develop an attitude of gratitude. The advice: Start saying "thank you." A simple "thank you" goes a long way with patients as well as with other staff members. Look for things to be thankful for, and soon you will see them multiply day by day.

# Chapter 15

# Helping patients sleep and eat

A cat eats and sleeps. Then maybe it plays with some string. A cat eats and sleeps. Then maybe it stretches. A cat eats and sleeps. Then maybe it curls up on your lap. A cat eats and sleeps.

If only our patients were cats, sleeping and eating without any concerns. Unfortunately, our patients are people. And many people suffer from two very common conditions: problems sleeping and problems eating. As a nurse, you need to have a tool kit of helpful hints and tricks to help your patients.

## Catch up on your zzz's

The normal sleep cycle is about one-and-a-half hours in length and includes passing through five stages of sleep: Stages 1, 2, 3, and 4 are sometimes called nonrapid eye movement sleep, and are followed by a period of rapid eye movement (REM) sleep.

Stages 1 and 2 are periods of light sleep during which eye movement, heart rate, and breathing slow down. Stages 3 and 4 are deeper periods of sleep. People awakened during theses stages often feel disoriented and groggy. It is the deeper stages of sleep—REM sleep—that refresh the body. It is a time when breaths quicken, the heart beats faster, muscles become immobile, and the person experiences vivid dreams.

### In search of some rest

People of all ages can experience trouble sleeping. Parents complain that babies and children have erratic sleep patterns; teens are notorious for staying up all night and wanting to sleep during the day; adults complain of not getting enough sleep; and older adults complain that they have trouble staying asleep.

## Sound sleep advice

Activities that help promote sleep are the same throughout a person's life-span. First, make sure your patients have careful and comprehensive assessments of their sleep problems. For example, if a person is having trouble sleeping because of allergies or enlarged tonsils and adenoids, these need to be addressed. People with restless leg syndrome or other limb movement disorders need to be evaluated and treated properly. Obstructive sleep apnea, a serious cause of sleep problems, also needs prompt attention.

Here is a list of hints that you can give your patients to help them sleep and feel rested in the morning:

- **Avoid stimulants.** Cutting caffeine at least four to six hours before bed-time can help a patient fall asleep easier. Caution them to avoid using alcohol as a sleep aid. Alcohol may initially help a person fall asleep, but it also causes disturbances in sleep resulting in less restful sleep. Restrict nicotine, as it too is a stimulant.

- **Relax before bedtime.** Provide time for quiet activities in the hour before bedtime. Try reading something light or doing some light stretching. Many nurses use aromatherapy for its relaxant effect, and commonly used essential oils include oils of chamomile, jasmine, lavender, neroli, rose, and marjoram. Add a few drops to a warm bath or sprinkle a few drops on a handkerchief or pillow. It is important to understand the difference between essential oils and fragrances. To learn more, review material in either *Clinical Aromatherapy: Holistic Nursing* by Ed Dossey et al., or *Clinical Aromatherapy 2004: Complementary & Alternative Medicine: A Research-Based Approach* by Ed Freeman.

- Other **bedtime relaxation rituals** that might work include asking the patient to gently wiggle his or her toes. You could also give him or her a head message, and/or ask the patient to apply lotion to his or her hands and feet.

- Provide for some **regular exercise** throughout the day to help your patients get a good night's sleep. Be aware that exercising in the evening may stimulate the patient too much and keep him or her awake.

- Provide for a **comfortable bedroom** situation. Keep the patient's bedroom as quiet, dark, and comfortable as tolerated. For many people, even the slightest noise or light can disturb sleep. Ear plugs and eye masks may help. Ideal room temperatures for sleeping are between 68°F and 72°F. Temperatures above 75°F or below about 54°F can disrupt sleep (Kryger et al.).

- **Eat right, sleep tight.** Help the patient to eat sensibly during the day and to avoid heavy meals before bedtime. Foods high in tryptophan, such as milk, can promote sleep. The patient can also try a bit of carbohydrate in the form of cereal or a banana, and should avoid overeating, as this may cause indigestion.

- Try tea. Some **herbal teas** such as kava kava, valerian, and chamomile have a reputation for aiding in sleep.

- Caution the patient to **avoid drinking fluids** after 8 p.m. Waking up to go to the bathroom may disrupt sleep and the patient may not be able to fall asleep again once disrupted.

- **Start a routine.** Do not allow the patient to nap during the day. Waking up at the same time in the morning helps develop a sleep rhythm.

## Just (help them) relax!

Progressive relaxation and relaxation breathing exercises can also aid in sleep. Progressive muscle relaxation (PMR) was described by Edmund Jacobson, MD, PhD, in the 1930s, and is based upon his premise that mental calmness is a natural result of physical relaxation. It is a deep relaxation technique that has been used to relieve insomnia as well as aid in the reduction of stress, anxiety, and pain. Simply stated, PMR is the practice of tensing (tightening) a muscle group and then releasing (relaxing) it, followed by moving on to another muscle group and repeating the process until you have systematically tensed and relaxed all muscles in the body.

Almost anyone can learn PMR. Usually it is best to start at the head or the feet. For example, start at the head and work down through all the body muscle groups, or start at the feet and work up to the head. Practicing relaxation breathing at the same time you practice PMR adds benefit.

Many people like to practice PMR in bed just before sleep, but it can be practiced in a sitting position as well. Sometimes PMR is a useful technique to use during long and tedious meetings.

 **Tip:** Here's how to start PMR:

1. Inhale and contract all your facial muscles, squeezing your eyes together, puckering up your mouth, and scrunching up your face. Now exhale and relax your facial muscles.

2. Inhale and tighten your neck muscles, and then exhale and release.

3. Inhale and contract your upper chest and upper back, and then exhale and release.

4. Inhale and contract the muscles in your left arm and hand, and then exhale and release.

5. Continue working your way through your body, contracting each muscle group and then releasing.

During PMR, keep your breath calm and do not hold it. Breathe in when contracting or tensing your muscles, and breathe out during release. As you practice this technique on your own or with your patients, gradually pay more attention to the release of body tension, as well as emotional tension.

## Relaxation or diaphragmatic breathing

Using the diaphragm and not the chest is the most efficient and relaxing way to breathe. Chest breathing elicits anxiety. Try it: Breathe only with your chest and see how you gradually become more and more anxious. Now, switch to breathing with your diaphragm, bringing in your breath through your nose, allowing it to slide through your chest without raising your chest, and continuing down to the area just above your navel. Some people have difficulty pushing out their abdominal area when inhaling and it may take some practice. But with practice, you and the patients you teach will find that it comes more naturally and that it results in a more alert and relaxed feeling.

 **Tip:** To practice diaphragmatic breathing, try the following:

1. Put one hand on your chest and the other on your abdominal area. Spread your fingers open, put the little finger near the navel, and put the thumb near the end of the sternum.

2.  Pay attention to your breathing. Breathe in slowly through your nose, allowing the breath to flow through the chest (keeping the hand over the chest still) and flow down toward the other hand, filling up the space under that hand.

3.  Continue to breathe in and blow up that space below the diaphragm like a big balloon.

4.  Now, exhale through the nose or mouth, sucking in the abdominal area to expel as much air as possible.

5.  Do not hold your breath, but continue with an inhalation through the nose again. Repeat this process for five to 10 minutes to feel a relaxation response.

### Caring for sleepwalkers

Most sleepwalkers are children, but occasionally a teen or adult will sleepwalk if he or she is sick, has a fever, is sleep deprived, or is under stress. Sleepwalkers tend to go back to bed on their own and don't usually remember sleepwalking. However, sometimes nurses need to prevent injury and help a sleepwalker move around obstacles in their way. Sometimes nurses may need to help them find their way back to their bed, especially if they are in unfamiliar surroundings. Sleepwalkers may startle easily, so it is best to guide them back to bed gently without waking them.

## "Hey, nurse, this food tastes lousy"

How many times have nurses heard that the food tastes lousy, or from more polite patients that it just doesn't taste the same? If you haven't yet, you will.

Some medications, such as certain antibiotics and antihypertensives; medications that cause dry mouth; treatments such as chemotherapy and radiation therapy; and certain disorders such as severe sinus infections, allergies, nasal polyps, and cancer, may cause a variety of appetite and taste problems. To help enhance a patient's appetite, make sure he or she has good oral hygiene before meals, remove any unpleasant smells or sights, and arrange the food in an attractive manner. In addition, working with the dietitian, you can try these tips to stimulate appetites and create a pleasant eating experience:

• Serve meat and poultry cold or at room temperature instead of piping hot. Substitute eggs if they taste better to the patient. Marinate meat or poultry in fruit juice, wine, vinegar-based salad dressing, or other sauces to enhance taste.

- Substitute fresh fruits and vegetables, pasta dishes, and milk products for meats if these taste better to the patient than meat.

- Offer fruit sorbet, sherbet, and fruit smoothies. Buy or make fruit juice popsicles.

- Peel carrots before eating or cooking, or try baby carrots to eliminate a bitter taste that some complain about.

- Use flavored mustards or horseradish as tolerated.

- Offer mouth rinses of fruit juice, wine, tea, ginger ale, club soda, or salted water before eating.

- Offer hard candy, such as lemon drops or mints, or gum.

- Experiment with spices and herbs. Perhaps spicier foods will be more enjoyable.

If the patient complains of a metallic taste, try these tips:

- Add something tart to the foods. Add orange, lime, or lemon juice, or citrus marmalades, to fruit salads and to sauces to add flavor to meats. Use vinegar, lemon juice, or pickles in creamy dressings for potato, macaroni, tuna, egg, or coleslaw salad.

- Avoid no-salt and low-salt varieties of canned soups or vegetables, unless the patient is on a sodium-restricted diet. Removing the salt tends to cause a metallic taste.

- Avoid using metal dishes and utensils. Try using plastic eating utensils, chopsticks, or porcelain Chinese soup spoons.

If the patient has a poor appetite or seems overwhelmed with the amount of food:

- Offer small amounts of food frequently

- Place small servings of food on small plates

- Cut sandwiches into smaller pieces

- Keep ready-to-eat snack foods such as pretzels, nuts, crackers, cookies, dried fruits, granola bars, and rice cakes handy

- Offer portable snacks such as cheese and crackers, muffins, ice cream, peanut butter, fruit, small boxes of raisins, and pudding as these may be more appealing than a meal

**Watch out:** Here are some things to avoid when dealing with patients and food:

- Do not force a patient to eat foods that taste bad. Instead, find substitutes.

- Avoid citrus juices (orange and grapefruit) immediately after brushing teeth with fluoride toothpaste because this can cause an unpleasant taste.

- Suggest that the patient reduce or stop smoking cigarettes because it interferes with taste.

- Talk with the patient about his or her alcohol use. Alcohol can cause dry mouth. Some alcoholic beverages, such as wine, can enhance appetite and taste. Overdrinking, however, interferes with taste.

## References

Gessel, A. H. (1989). "Edmund Jacobson, MD, PhD: The founder of scientific relaxation." *Int J Psychosomatics*. 36(1-4): 5–14.

Kryger, M., T. Roth, and W. Dement (2005). *Principles and Practice of Sleep Medicine*, 4th edition. Philadelphia: WB Saunders.

"Managing Eating Problems: 'Food Just Doesn't Taste the Same.' " University of Michigan. Available at *www.cancer.med.umich.edu/learn/nutrtastesame.htm*. Accessed June 10, 2007.

National Sleep Foundation. Available at *www.sleepfoundation.org*. Accessed June 6, 2007.

"When Food Doesn't Taste Good." University of Pittsburgh Medical Center. Available at *www.upmc.com/HealthManagement/ManagingYourHealth/PersonalHealth/Men/?chunkiid=13965*. Accessed June 10, 2007.

# Chapter 16

# Handling anger and violence

Everyone encounters angry people. And everyone gets angry from time to time. Patients get angry. Nurses get angry. Everyone "loses his or her cool" from time to time. It may be uncomfortable to handle anger, but it is a necessary task. And dealing with anger or other emotions can often strengthen and enrich a relationship.

## The anatomy of anger

Anger is an emotion—nothing more and nothing less. It's a *very powerful* emotion that can stem from feelings of frustration, hurt, annoyance, or disappointment. It is a normal human emotion that can range from slight irritation to strong rage.

Sometimes anger can even be a good thing. When people are treated unfairly, anger can motivate them to do something about their situation and stand up for themselves. The hard part about anger is learning what to do with these strong feelings, and how to handle these strong feelings in others.

However, most of the time, anger does not stand alone. There is usually a catalyst for anger—sometimes it is a situation, but most often it is another feeling. In order to handle anger effectively, we need to find out what that other feeling or catalyst is. So, part of handling anger is finding out what is behind the anger. We need to ask ourselves one question when we feel angry, and find out the answer to the same question from our patients when they get angry: What feeling did you experience first, just before the anger?

## What makes our patients angry?

Patients often get angry when they:

- Become frustrated, don't know what to expect, or experience a culture shock in the healthcare arena

- Are afraid of the diagnosis, treatments needed, and/or outcomes of care

- Don't get their way, or have a feeling of loss of personal control

- Feel overlooked, such as when they are not included in their care-planning discussions

- Are discouraged with themselves when they don't understand something, think they could have done something better, and/or are not getting better as fast as they had hoped

Feel free to add some other examples from your own experience.

### How can I tell when a patient is angry?

Here are some common anger signals. Look for these signs and you might be able to address the anger (or the feeling behind the anger) before the patient acts out his or her anger inappropriately:

- Stomping away or acting short

- Becoming quiet and not talking

- Breathing faster, becoming red in the face

- Clenching teeth, making fists, tensing other muscles

- Complaining of headache or stomachache

 **Watch out:** Don't let anger (or that other feeling behind the anger) control the situation.

Don't let an angry patient control you. Don't let an angry situation control you. Take charge of the situation. Learn how to release your anger in safe ways, and/or handle situations and the feelings that happen just before the anger, in effective ways. Otherwise, you'll be like a tightly wound top that spins out of control, rather than a graceful dancer releasing your energy in a more controlled way.

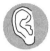

**Listen up:** Janet, a patient, explained that anger is like hot lava coming out of a volcano. It can either come out slowly and controlled, thereby not hurting anyone and giving people time to move out of the way, or it can get trapped underneath the volcano and gain such momentum and strength that it blows the top off the volcano and spews out everywhere and over everything. This kind of anger, she said, is the destructive and hurtful kind. So, another way to look at handling anger in ourselves and others is to help the lava flow rather than explode and spew.

## Let's go behind the anger

Getting in touch with the feeling behind the anger is sometimes tricky. But it gets easier with practice.

**Tip:** The next time you get angry, stop yourself and take three breaths, and then ask yourself what is going on that has made you angry.

Are you angry because you feel you cannot do your best in a given situation? If so, perhaps frustration is the feeling behind the anger. Are you angry because you overheard some of your colleagues talking about going out after work and you were not invited? Perhaps the feeling behind the anger is a feeling of being left out or overlooked. Are you angry because, once again, someone important to you has not lived up to the agreement he or she made with you? Perhaps the feeling behind the anger is feeling let down.

Once you get to the feeling behind the anger, then choose a way to deal with that feeling. How do you deal with frustration? Ask yourself whether your expectations are too high. Are you trying to accomplish too much? Are you forgetting to ask for help? How do you deal with feeling left out? How do you deal with feeling let down? As you can see, dealing with these feelings behind the anger is much different from dealing with pure anger.

Once you have practiced this yourself and are getting the hang of it, start using it with patients (and colleagues too). When a patient is angry, finding out the feeling behind the anger helps you to determine the real problem, problem-solve the situation, and, once discovered, make the situation easier to handle.

### Determining the feeling behind the anger

Try saying something like this to the patient: "I know that you are angry right now. I would like to help you. First, I need to know more about the situation. Can you tell me exactly what happened to make you feel the way you are feeling now?"

Doing this helps in a variety of ways. First, it lets the patient know you care. Second, by giving you details about what has made him or her angry, it brings the patient into a rational thinking mode rather than an emotional thinking mode. And third, it helps you begin to figure out what you think might be the feeling behind the anger.

In a gentle manner, make sure you get enough information so that you can understand it. Make sure that the patient has enough time to respond to your questions without interruption.

While telling you his or her story, ask the person to look up when talking rather than look down. Looking down keeps the person in an emotional state. Looking up moves him or her into a rational thinking state, preparing the mind for problem solving.

### Use active listening

Active listening is paying attention to what the other person doesn't say, as well as what he or she is saying. Active listening is a way of listening without getting tangled up in your own emotions. Active listening has also been called:

- Listening with the third ear

- Listening with curiosity

- Listening to learn the "whys" of the situation

- Listening to understand

Learning the "whys" through active listening doesn't mean to ask "why" questions, because this often makes matters worse. So, avoid questions such as "*Why* did you do that?" and "*Why* didn't you talk to me about this before?" Directly asking a question beginning with the word "why" can make the person defensive.

Instead, ask the person to tell you in detail "what" happened to cause him or her to be angry.

Then, repeat what you think you heard. In this way, you will show interest and will start to get to the real problem. Ask the patient if you got it right. Say something like "Sir, let me see if I got it: You are upset because the tech brought in your tray and did not help set up your meal. You want more attention around mealtime because you can't do things for yourself." Doing something like this helps you build a connection with the patient, shows the patient that you were listening, and helps you determine the feeling behind the anger, which in this case seems to be a frustration in the person's inability to care for him or herself.

Now, you and the patient can solve this problem of the tray and the meal. It may not prevent the situation from happening again, and it may not address all the feelings behind the anger, but it is a start and it is building a bridge of trust and cooperation. You've changed the dynamic. You've made it clear which side of the discussion you're on—the patient's side.

## Empathy goes a long way

An integral part of handling a patient's anger is letting the person know you understand the story, letting him or her know that you get it, or showing the person that you empathize with him or her. Recall that empathy means you recognize, perceive, and directly connect with the emotion of another. It is different from sympathy, which means you feel bad because of another person's situation. Empathy is patient-centered. Sympathy is you-centered. Make sure your responses take the patient into consideration. Keep your tone even.

In addition to those empathy dos, make sure you avoid these empathy don'ts:

- Don't be condescending

- Don't pretend to understand something that doesn't make sense to you

- Don't give unsolicited advice

- Don't respond with a cliché that dismisses how the person feels

- Don't jump to conclusions

### Work out a solution

Working out a solution does not mean telling patients how you would deal with it if you were in their situation. You can certainly offer choices. But often, hearing them out and showing empathy for what they are going through will help them to calm themselves down enough to work out a solution by themselves, or at least get them started in that direction. Your role as an active listener is to help the person you are talking with to recognize the source of his or her negative feeling. Your job is also to help them problem-solve for themselves. Ask them questions like "I see what you are saying now. I think I understand your dilemma. Do you have any ideas of how to solve this (What will need to happen for you to be happy? How to handle this? What will soothe you?)?

## Tip time: How to handle angry situations

**Tip:** Don't waste a lot of time, emotion, and energy trying to solve a problem that's not solvable. If a problem is not solvable, admit it. Say something like "This situation is out of our control. What we can control is . . ." Then, offer something that you can do to help the situation even if only indirectly.

**Tip:** Do not allow yourself to get into a heated battle with the patient. There are many tricks to this. One way is to speak softly and slowly. Some nurses even just mouth words so that nothing can be heard. Patients often quiet down because they want to hear how you might be able to help them.

**Tip:** Avoid saying things like "calm down," and avoid touching the person. Even though you mean to soothe the situation by doing these things, it often inflames it.

**Tip:** Avoid escalating the situation—go one down, not one up. Going one up means that you try to outmaneuver the patient. Then, the patient tries to one-up you, and the situation just escalates higher and higher. To stop the conflict from escalating, go one down, or make a conciliatory remark. You can say something like "You are right. It is extremely noisy in here. No wonder you can't rest." Or "Gee, I am late (even if you are only one minute later than the patient expected you). But I am here now." A bit of levity, but not flippancy, and being patient-focused might turn things around quickly.

**Tip:** Avoid excuses or explanations, such as "Everyone is so busy," "We don't have enough staff members," or "There are sicker patients than you." No one really wants to hear all that. They just want to know when their needs are going to be addressed.

 **Tip:** Call for help if the situation seems unmanageable.

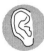 **Listen up:** Tim, a psychiatric consultant in a general hospital, was called to help the staff deal with "a totally crazy woman" who was not doing anything the staff wanted her to do. She was throwing things and screaming at them, and appeared to be ungrateful that the staff saved her life. The staff needed Tim to "straighten her out." Upon interviewing the patient, Tim found out that she was indeed grateful for being alive, but that was overshadowed by the total shock she experienced when she saw the incision that went from her navel to her pubic bone. The patient explained that she was well known in her neighborhood for being in her garden in the summer in a bikini. As she talked, Tim grew to understand her further. She received her recognition in life from her beautiful garden and her vast collection of bikinis. What Tim's personal value system might say about her was not relevant to her care. What was relevant was that her impression of the result of the surgery, her self-esteem, and her self-identity were in jeopardy. Toward the end of the discussion, Tim mentioned to her that he knew the nurses caring for her were experts in scar care and would be happy to give her guidance on how to minimize the appearance of her scar. That was all it took. Tim informed the nurses of the blow to her self-esteem and self-identity, and suggested that they approach her with the goal of scar minimization. It worked: The "bikini queen" did everything asked of her, the nurses were happy, and she was happy.

 **Listen up:** Here's a thought question: What was the feeling behind the anger for the "bikini queen"?

 **Tip:** Sometimes people are beyond frustration, and are upset, angry, or furious. Always call for help and institute your facility's safety plan if you suspect that the patient will become violent.

 **Tip:** Here are some hints for handling a patient who seems frustrated, angry, and on the way to becoming violent:

- Avoid threatening behaviors. Threatening behaviors may increase fear or prompt assault.

- Avoid shouting. If the person is not listening to you, raising your voice may not help. A person with schizophrenia may be preoccupied with inner voices (auditory hallucinations).

- Avoid criticizing. This might escalate the situation.

- Avoid baiting the patient. Don't do anything to encourage wild or impulsive behavior.

- Avoid standing over the patient. Keep a comfortable distance and put yourself at the same level as the patient. If he or she is seated, seat yourself.

- Avoid eye contact or touching. This might be perceived as threatening.

- Give the patient some sense of control combined with a sense of safety. Often, the presence of others is reassuring.

- Don't back yourself or the patient into a corner.

## References

"Dealing with Anger." KidsHealth. Available at *www.kidshealth.org/kid/feeling/emotion/anger.html*. Accessed June 9, 2007.

Godin, S. "How to deal with an angry customer." Posted September 14, 2006. Available at *http://sethgodin.typepad.com/seths_blog/2006/09/how_to_deal_wit.html*. Accessed June 10, 2007.

Ho, B. C., et al. (2003). "Schizophrenia and other psychotic disorders." *Textbook of Clinical Psychiatry*, 4th edition. Washington, DC: American Psychiatric Publishing.

"Mental Health: Managing Anger." WebMD. *Available at http://men.webmd.com/guide/anger-management*. Accessed June 10, 2007.

# Chapter 17

# Dealing with suicidal behaviors

 **Tip:** All nurses need to feel comfortable completing a suicide assessment.

Many nurses don't feel comfortable completing a suicide assessment. Some nurses can't imagine anyone thinking that killing him or herself is the best solution to any problem. However, many of the patients we serve have thought that way and some are actively suicidal, and we are not even aware of it. Being aware of the signs of suicide, and making a suicide assessment, can save your patient's life. As with many other assessments, practice facilitates mastery. This chapter will give you lots of guidelines and tips to help.

It is important to remember that most suicide attempts are expressions of extreme distress, not harmless bids for attention. Also, any person who has expressed suicidal ideation should not be left alone and needs immediate treatment.

## What if I think someone is suicidal?

One way to determine whether a person is thinking about suicide is to ask directly: "Are you thinking about suicide? Are you planning to kill yourself?" Doing this will not plant thoughts in the person's head. Doing this will not cause the person to consider suicide if he or she was not thinking about it. Doing this will not cause the person to try suicide. By asking directly, you show you are not afraid to tackle the hardest of situations, and it is a way to show the patient that you can be trusted. Suicidal individuals seek out those whom they trust and feel connected to in some way. One of the most important factors in preventing a suicide is the presence of a supportive person.

If it is hard to be so direct, you can try a less direct approach. You can say, "Many people in your situation may have thought that life would not be worth living: Have you ever had these thoughts?" or "Many people in your situation may have thought that they would be better off dead: Has this thought ever occurred to you?" This opens the door for further, more direct assessment. It also tells the patient you know this happens and that he or she is not alone in his or her thinking.

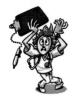

**Don't panic:** If a person does tell you that he or she is suicidal, here's what you can do:

- Stay calm and listen.

- Let the person talk about his or her feelings.

- Be accepting, and do not judge.

- Ask whether the person has a plan, and if so, what it is.

- Don't swear secrecy.

- Do not leave the patient alone. Take him or her with you if you must, so you can get help.

## Some facts and stats

In 2004, suicide was the eleventh leading cause of death in the United States, accounting for 32,439 deaths. The overall rate was 10.9 suicide deaths per 100,000 people. Suicidal behavior is complex. Some risk factors vary with age, gender, or ethnic group and may occur in combination or change over time (Numbers, NIMH).

Here are some more facts and figures for you:

- Suicide is the eighth leading cause of death for males.

- Suicide is the sixteenth leading cause of death for females.

- Almost four times as many males as females die by suicide. More than four times as many males as females age 20–24 die by suicide.

- Firearms, suffocation, and poison are by far the most common methods of suicide.

Suicide deaths by age group are as follows:

- Children (10–14 years old): 1.3 for every 100,000.

- Adolescents (15–19 years old): 8.2 for every 100,000.

- Young adults (20–24 years old): 12.5 for every 100,000.

- Older adults (65 years and older): 14.3 for every 100,000. Non-Hispanic white men age 85 or older had an even higher rate, with 17.8 suicide deaths for every 100,000 (Numbers, NIMH).

## Don't ignore the warning signs

All mentions of suicide must be taken seriously. Warning signs include:

- Thoughts or talk of death or suicide

- Thoughts or talk of self-harm or harm to others

- Aggressive behavior or impulsiveness

- Previous suicide attempts, which increases the risk for future suicide attempts and completed suicide

### Assessing the possibility of suicidal thoughts

Ask the patient the following questions to assess the possibility of suicidal thoughts:

- You have been through a lot lately: How has that affected your energy (appetite, ability to sleep)?

- Many people in your situation may feel sad and blue or depressed: Do you feel that way?

- Have you ever felt so sad and blue that you thought that maybe life was not worth living?

- You have been in a lot of pain lately: Have you ever wished you could go to sleep and just not wake up?

- Have you been thinking a lot about death recently?

- Have you recently thought about harming yourself or killing yourself?

- Have things ever reached the point that you've thought of harming yourself?

If the person says that he or she has thought about self-harm or suicide, the next step is to assess whether the person has a plan and the ability to carry out the plan. Ask questions such as these:

- Have you made a specific plan to harm (kill) yourself? If so, what is it?

- Do you have a gun (knife) available for your use? (Find out if the person has access to accomplish the plan.)

- What preparations have you made? (This might include purchasing specific items, writing a note or a will, making financial arrangements, taking steps to avoid being found, and/or practicing the plan.)

- Have you spoken to anyone about your plans?

- Would you be able to tell someone if you were about to harm (kill) yourself?

## Keeping the patient safe

Your next step is to make sure the patient is safe. Most facilities have policies about levels of observation or supervision for patients who are a suicidal risk. There is also a process for further assessment of the patient. Again, never leave a person who has expressed suicidal thoughts alone. Take him or her with you to get help. Always read and follow your facility's policies.

In general, there are some universal safety measures to take with a person who is suicidal:

- Keep the person on continuous observation, such as 1:1 or in your line of sight.

- Restrict the person's environment for safety. Ask the person to remain in a certain area where staff members can see him or her at all times.

- Do not allow the person to be alone in a room.

- Check the person at intervals of five, 15, or 30 minutes.

- Staff supervision is necessary when a patient uses items such as sharps (nail cutters, razors, or scissors), cigarettes, and/or matches; is around potential poisons, such as cleaning supplies; uses the bathroom or kitchen; and/or goes off the unit for treatments, therapies, or tests.

## Special consideration for children and teens

Children and teens who are suicidal report feelings of depression, anger, anxiety, hopelessness, and worthlessness. They feel helpless to change frustrating circumstances or to find a solution for their problems. In addition to depression, family conflicts and suicidal death of a relative, friend, or acquaintance are risk factors for suicide among children and teens. In the case of another person's suicide, children or teens may need intervention to prevent feelings of guilt, trauma, or social isolation.

Danger signs that a teen may be considering suicide include:

- Undergoing a dramatic personality change

- Giving away prized possessions

- Writing notes or poems about death

- Talking about suicide, even jokingly

- Making comments such as "I can't take it anymore" or "I won't be a problem for you much longer"

- Previously attempting suicide

- Running away from home

- Having other symptoms or risk factors for depression, such as difficulty getting along with parents and friends, difficulty in school, or acting bored or withdrawn (American Academy of Child & Adolescent Psychiatry)

Some approaches to prevent suicide include establishing telephone crisis hotlines; restricting access to suicide methods (e.g., firearms); counseling to reduce "copycat" suicides, especially for youth; screening for risk factors of suicide; and training professionals to improve recognition and treatment of mood disorders and other situations that might lead to suicide.

**Don't forget:** Share the National Suicide Prevention Lifeline with your patients. The National Suicide Prevention Lifeline is a service available to anyone. You may call for yourself or for someone you care about. All calls are confidential. The toll-free number, available 24/7, is 800/273-TALK (8255).

## References

"Facts for Families: Teen Suicide." American Academy of Child & Adolescent Psychiatry. Available at *http://aacap.org/page.ww?section=Facts+for+Families &name=Teen+Suicide*. Accessed June 2, 2007.

Jacobs, D., et al. (2003). "Practice Guideline for the Assessment and Treatment of Patients with Suicidal Behaviors." American Psychiatric Association. Available at *www.psych.org/psych_pract/treatg/pg/SuicidalBehavior_ 05-15-06.pdf*. Accessed June 2, 2007.

"Suicide in the U.S.: Statistics and Prevention." National Institute of Mental Health. Available at *www.nimh.nih.gov/publicat/harmsway.cfm*. Accessed June 2, 2007.

"The Numbers Count: Mental Disorders in America." National Institute of Mental Health. Available at *www.nimh.nih.gov/publicat/numbers.cfm*. Accessed June 2, 2007.

# Part Three

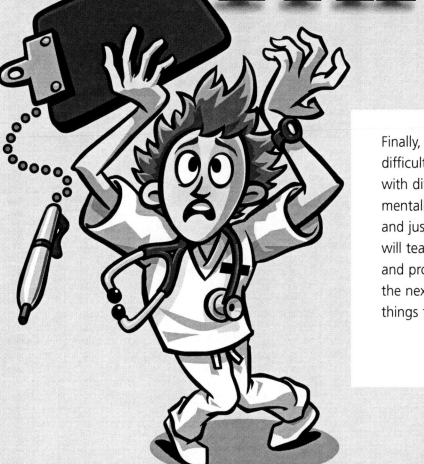

Finally, let's focus on the most difficult patient—you. Working with difficult patients can leave you mentally exhausted, physically tired, and just plain stressed. This section will teach you to care for yourself and provide some inspiration for the next time you need to see things from another point of view.

# Chapter 18

# Finding ways to handle your stress

*Old Nurse Hubbard*
*went to her cupboard*
*to refuel her tired body and brain.*
*When she got there*
*the cupboard was bare,*
*so poor Nurse Hubbard stayed tired and drained.*

Nursing is known as the caring profession. Nurses are known as caring individuals. Caring and anticipating needs are strengths of those in nursing. They are our best assets, and the assets most recognized by others.

But our greatest assets can also be our worst liabilities. In other words, caring has two sides to it: Caring for others is noble and fulfilling, but caring too much, or using up all of our energy caring without caring for ourselves, can leave us tired and drained.

How many of us have gone to our cupboards to find them bare?

Those of us who continually have bare cupboards face burnout, physical stress, and increasing emotional stress. Some of us may become sicker than our patients. Being low on emotional fuel can enhance any emotional struggles that may come up in our work. Then, we need more energy to cope, and the cumulative effect can start to grow out of control. Nurses are jeopardizing their future success as nurses, and their ability to advance their careers in nursing, by giving too much without stopping to refuel.

The daily work of nursing is stressful emotionally, physically, and spiritually. One might say that nurses, because of the type of work we do, need to pamper ourselves and be pampered by others more than those in other lines of work. However, what do we find ourselves doing when we are not at work? Often, we are taking care of children, aging parents, sick relatives, or ill neighbors; volunteering at soup kitchens; grocery shopping; carpooling; and performing many other seemingly endless errands. Or, sadly, for some of us, we turn to maladaptive methods of coping and drink alcohol to excess or take drugs to medicate against the emotional and physical pain our work brings.

## Caring for the most difficult patient: yourself

In order to take care of challenging patients, we need to make time to take care of ourselves. Nurses who do not take care of their own health needs are often the ones most likely to have problems caring for challenging patients. We need to face up to the reality that spending our work life caring for others is a heavy burden, and we must take some time to recharge, and refill our cupboards. We need to address the emotional toll our work takes on us.

### Stress creates wear and tear on the body
Stress can be emotional, physical, or spiritual. The first step in handling stress is to make sure that we understand how we cope with stress.

As nurses, we can make the assumption that our personal life and our work life cause us stress. There is really no need to make a list of our stressors— this might cause us more stress. But it's safe to assume that we have stress. We have all developed methods to handle our stress: Sometimes we develop adaptive ways and other times we use maladaptive methods. Start by listing some coping methods and separating them into those that help and those that hinder you. Then do more of what helps, and systematically eliminate or change those that hinder. Use this chart to help:

## Figure 4: Assessing your coping style

| Coping Mechanisms That Help Me | Coping Mechanisms That Hinder Me |
|---|---|
| Yoga class once a week | Being silent when I don't like what someone has said to me |
| Talking with my older brother about my work life | Complaining and gossiping about other people at work |
| | |
| | |
| | |
| | |

Let's take a look at some concepts to help us to handle stress better and to fill up our cupboards.

## Stress relief 101

Sometimes the way we look at things causes us increased stress. Here are some ways of thinking that add to stress. Do any of these ring true for you?

- **Extreme thinking:** Sometimes we see things with no middle ground or no gray. It is all black and white, all or nothing, good or bad.

- **Overgeneralizing/blowing things out of proportion:** Everything is a crisis. "*No one* here knows what he or she is doing." "I *never* get a good assignment."

- **Mind reading/fortune-telling:** You predict the future in a negative way: "This is going to be another rotten day."

- **Jumping to conclusions without enough evidence or guessing about what other people are thinking about us:** "*They* don't know what it is like to work on the floor. This is just one more thing they thought up to make our days difficult."

- **Personalizing:** Jumping to a conclusion that something is directly connected to you: "Everyone knows I've been off work because I can't cope."

## Make a pact with yourself

One way to reduce your stress is to change the way you look at things. Try these alternatives and see how they work for you:

- Change extreme thinking into reality thinking. Look for the gray between the black and white.

- Stop overgeneralizing and recognize that what is happening now is only what is happening now. Nothing lasts forever. Look for times when good things happen to you, such as when you do get a good assignment.

- Stop mind reading. Ask for clarification and details. Check out the facts. What does the policy say? What does the procedure mandate?

- Gather your data before making a conclusion. We all know we need to make a comprehensive patient assessment before a diagnosis can be made. Use the same principles when coming to a conclusion (diagnosis) about a situation that has caused you discomfort.

- Come to grips with the reality that the world doesn't revolve around you. Yes, sorry to say, most of the time other people are so concerned about themselves that they don't even think about how their actions might affect you.

## Use The Four Agreements™

The Four Agreements offers nurses simple, brief, and concise wisdom that can aid us in our daily lives. Making these four agreements with yourself is one way to reduce your stress and replenish your emotional cupboard:

1. **Be impeccable with your word.** Speak with conviction and integrity. Avoid gossiping about others.

2. **Don't take anything personally.** Remember that what others say and do is a projection of their own reality. It is not about you.

3. **Don't make assumptions.** Ask questions to determine what is behind what is going on. Ask questions and express what you really want. Communicate as clearly as you can.

4. **Always do your best.** Strive to always do your best, and when you don't do as well as you hoped, avoid negative self-judgment, self-abuse, and regret. Your best may not always be "A" work, but it will be the best you can offer at that moment.

## Change stress into relief

In her article "Break the cycle of stress with PBR3," Becky Graner, MS, RN, IAC, shares a simple tool that aids in stress relief. PBR3 stands for pause, breathe, relax, reflect, rewrite. Let's see how it works. Adhere to the process in the following table the next time you are in a stressful situation at work, or just before going in to take care of a patient who presents a challenge to you.

### Figure 5: Finding relief from stress

| | |
|---|---|
| **Pause** | Simply stop thinking. You can continue doing something such as walking down the hall, washing your hands, or another activity that has become automatic for you. Simply stop your thoughts. |
| **Breathe** | Stop the chatter in your mind by paying attention to your breathing. Just focus on your breaths and count, say a prayer, or repeat an affirmation to yourself. Don't try to control your breath. And don't hold your breath. |
| **Relax** | Simply taking a pause and a few breaths, particularly diaphragmatic breathing (see Chapter 15), takes you out of a reactive state and into a more relaxed state. When you are relaxed, your thinking will clear. |
| **Reflect** | Debrief yourself. What was going on that led up to the situation that bothered you? If you felt angry, what was the feeling behind the anger? Was your response out of proportion to the situation? Were you thinking the worst? |
| **Rewrite** | Check yourself to find out where you may have been taking things too personally, making assumptions, or doing some of the other automatic thinking processes that cause more stress than not. Rethink or rewrite these into more realistic assumptions. Using humor, empathy, or compassion may soothe you. |

*Source: Based on Becky Graner's "Break the cycle of stress with PBR3"*

## Take a lesson from our friends from "down under"

And lastly, take a look at this list of things that nurses can do to help reduce stress, written by fours nurses from New South Wales, Australia. Use them to help keep yourself focused:

- Keep things in perspective.

- Talk about what bothers you with family and friends.

- Find out as much as you can about a situation that bothers you.

- Ease up on yourself.

- Stop wasting time worrying. Confront your problems and make plans to solve them.

- Set realistic goals.

- Take care of yourself physically. Exercise regularly and eat right.

- Learn some form of relaxation and practice it regularly.

- Make sure there is plenty of fun in your life.

- Remember that everyone slides back every once in a while (Brunero et al.).

## References

Brunero, S., D. Cowan, A. Grochulski, and A. Garvey. "Stress Management for Nurses." Available at *www.nswnurses.asn.au/multiattachments/5695/DocumentName/Nurses_Stress_Management_Booklet.pdf*. Accessed June 9, 2007.

Graner, B. "Break the cycle of stress with PBR3." *American Nurse Today*, (2)5:56–57.

Kenney, E. "Creating fulfillment in today's workplace: A guide for nurses." *American Journal of Nursing*, 98 (5):44–48.

Ruiz, D. M. (1997). *The Four Agreements: A Practical Guide to Personal Freedom (A Toltec Wisdom Book)*. San Rafael, CA: Amber-Allen Publishing.

Selye, H. (1956). *The Stress of Life*. New York: McGraw-Hill.

"The Four Agreements." The Toltec teachings of Don Miguel Ruiz and Don Jose Ruiz. Available at *www.miguelruiz.com/fouragreements.html*. Accessed June 9, 2007.

# Chapter 19

# A lesson from the past creates a brighter future

Sometimes our most challenging or difficult patients teach us the most. Here's a story from a nurse who graduated in 1950. She still remembers this challenging patient from her nursing school days, working in a large, inner-city hospital. Here is her story.

## Listening to Walter

I was scared of Walter, a huge, battered-looking man with far advanced tuberculosis (TB), who glared at me with bloodshot eyes and resisted my efforts to comfort him.

"You don't know what you are doing," he informed me, coughing up a huge blob of blood-tinged sputum.

"At least let me give you mouth care," I replied, holding a sputum cup and wiping off his face.

He agreed. As I started to do mouth care, I was alarmed to see skin sloughing from his gums, which oozed bright red serum.

"How long have your gums been bleeding?" I asked.

"Ain't no bleeding. You see any blood? You don't know what you are doing and you don't know what you are seeing!"

Somehow, I got through the rest of Walter's care.

Later, when I told the head nurse about Walter's gums, I found out that Walter was getting an experimental medication for TB and it was determined that he was having a reaction to it that caused his skin to peel from his gums. It got worse. The reaction progressed as layers of skin all over his body began to slough. The medication was stopped and various treatments were tried, but nothing stopped the shedding of dermis and the subsequent oozing of blood and serum. It was impossible to touch Walter without removing some of his skin. His sheets were a mess and his room stank. He got worse and worse, coughing and spitting and cursing at me.

I dreaded going into Walter's room, but found him on my patient list nearly every morning. One day, glad to have a little help, I took a first-year nursing student in with me. By this time, I was more adept at caring for Walter and less intimidated by his belligerence. But he was too much for the neophyte, who started to faint. I had to get her out of the room so I could finish Walter's care.

"Why do you bring these dumb people in here? They don't know what they are doing either," Walter complained loudly.

I was glad when that rotation ended and I no longer had to care for Walter. But a few weeks later, I found myself back in his room, as I was providing supper relief for the other nurses. The charge nurse informed me that Walter was not expected to live much longer. I found him emaciated and breathing with difficulty, but his red eyes still glared ferociously.

"How come you are back?" he asked.

"Supper relief. I won't stay long. I just need to see how much you ate today," I answered.

"Never mind that stuff. Sit down here and listen to me," he demanded.

He looked so troubled, I sat down. Walter told me rambling, incoherent stories of his life—a kaleidoscope of bar brawls, sleeping in gutters, getting in street fights, going to jail, and watching other men get killed. Several times, he stopped, shook his head, and said, "What these eyes have seen."

I could not always make out the words, but sensed he was desperate to have his life and suffering remembered. He rambled on for quite some time. I sat and listened. He had been in isolation and never had a visitor the entire time he was in the hospital. Finally, Walter lay back on his pillow, exhausted. Then, he closed his eyes, seemed more relaxed than ever, and went to sleep.

I tiptoed out of the room. The charge nurse was not very happy with me for spending so much time with Walter. But I felt it was the best nursing job I'd ever done. Walter died peacefully the following morning.

Walter taught me more than any instructor or textbook. Beneath his repulsive appearance and manner, Walter showed me that we all share a common humanity. We are all human beings struggling to make sense of our lives. Walter was literally dying to be heard. Nursing often seems to be a matter of tearing around to get things done, but our efficiency may take us away from people who need us most. For our sake, as well as theirs, let's slow down and take the time to listen. In recognizing patients as human beings, we affirm our own humanity as well.

—*Special thanks to Betty Scher, RN, for sharing this story written by her classmate, Mildred E. Barnard, RN, The Johns Hopkins Hospital School of Nursing, Class of 1950.*

# Glossary

## A

**Active listening**—Paying attention to what the other person doesn't say, as well as to what he or she is saying.

**Amygdala**—An almond-shaped structure deep in the brain that is believed to be a communication hub between the parts of the brain that process incoming sensory signals and the parts that interpret these signals.

**Axon terminals** (also known as **presynaptic terminals**)—Fine branches that have specialized swellings that end near the dendrites of another neuron.

## C

**Compulsions**—Acts that a person performs as a way to deal with obsessive thoughts.

**Conscious mind**—Part of Freud's iceberg model, it is what we are aware of at any particular moment: our present perceptions, memories, thoughts, fantasies, and feelings.

**Crazy**—A term that can mean a multitude of things—anything from madness and insanity, to wild enthusiasm (the crowd went crazy), to some degree of fondness (he was crazy about her).

**Culture shock**—Anxiety produced when a person moves into a completely new environment.

# D

**Delirium**—A term used to describe an acute psychotic state, with rapid onset, caused by an agent or condition that when removed or treated will result in the resolution of the psychotic state.

**Delusions**—False personal beliefs that are not part of the person's culture and do not change, even when other people present proof that the beliefs are not true or logical.

**Delusions of grandeur**—False personal beliefs that occur when people think they are famous historical figures.

**Drug addiction**—A chronic disease that is characterized by compulsive drug seeking and use, despite harmful consequences.

# E

**Ego**—In Freud's view, the part of the mind that is the problem solver. The ego understands that other people have needs and desires too, and that sometimes being impulsive or selfish, as the id wants to be, can hurt us in the long run.

**Ego defense mechanisms**—Those things that unconsciously block or distort our thoughts and beliefs into more acceptable, less threatening ones.

# G

**Generalized anxiety disorder (GAD)**—Excessive, unrealistic worry that lasts for more than six months. Physical symptoms include trembling, insomnia, dizziness, and irritability.

**H**

Hallucinations—Tricks of the mind that are perceived as real by the person having them, but not by others. Hallucinations come in many varieties, including auditory, visual, olfactory, gustatory, and tactile.

Hippocampus—The part of the brain that encodes threatening events into memories.

Hypnagogic hallucinations—Unusual sensory experiences or thoughts that occur when a person is falling asleep.

Hypnopompic hallucinations—Unusual sensory experiences or thoughts that occur when waking up from sleep.

**I**

Id—In Freud's view, the part of the mind that is sensitive to our needs (hunger, thirst, avoidance of pain, and desire for sex), and strives to keep us in a state of satisfaction or pleasure.

Insane—A legal term meaning that the person has a mental illness of such a severe nature that he or she cannot distinguish fantasy from reality, cannot conduct his or her affairs, or is subject to uncontrollable impulsive behavior.

**N**

Neuron—The basic functional unit of the brain.

Neuronal axon—The part of the neuron that carries messages away from the cell body, relaying these messages to other cells.

Neuronal dendrites—Extending from the cell body, they branch out and serve as the main apparatus for receiving input from other nerve cells.

# O

Obsessions—Thoughts that occur over and over again.

Obsessive-compulsive disorder (OCD)—Characterized by persistent, recurring thoughts that exaggerate anxiety or fears; the need to do something (compulsion) to rid oneself of the recurring thought (obsession).

# P

Panic disorder—Severe distress that causes the individual to believe he or she is having a health problem (such as a heart attack) or will lose control.

Paranoia—The presence of extreme fears usually associated with a disorder of thought.

Paranoid delusions—False personal beliefs that someone is being deliberately cheated on, harassed, poisoned, spied on, or plotted against by the people they care about.

Personality disorder—When a person has such deeply rooted personality traits that he or she becomes inflexible and cannot adjust his or her approach when it is needed.

Post-traumatic stress disorder (PTSD)—A cluster of symptoms that persist after experiencing a traumatic event (war, sexual or physical assault, unexpected death of a loved one, disaster).

Preconscious mind—Part of Freud's iceberg model, it contains those things that are not in our awareness all of the time, but that can be brought into our awareness easily.

Progressive muscle relaxation—The practice of tensing (tightening) a muscle group and then releasing (relaxing) it, followed by moving on to another muscle group and repeating the process until you have systematically tensed and relaxed all muscles in the body.

Psychosis—A generic psychiatric term for a mental state often described as involving a loss of contact with reality.

# S

**Schizoaffective disorder**—When a person has the symptoms of schizophrenia combined with symptoms of either mania or depression or both.

**Schizoid personality disorder**—When a person appears aloof and displays little or no emotion.

**Schizophrenia**—A neuropsychiatric condition (disorder of the brain) that is both a thought disorder and an emotional disorder.

**Schizotypal personality disorder**—When a person has difficulty developing close relationships with other people, and may have delusions and other unusual behaviors.

**Social anxiety disorder**—An individual's extreme anxiety that he or she is being judged by others or a belief that he or she is behaving in a way that might cause embarrassment.

**Superego**—In Freud's view, the part of the mind that is sometimes called the internal parent. The superego is forever making judgments regarding what we have done right or wrong.

**Synapse**—An electrical/chemical interchange in the intercellular space between the presynaptic neuron (the cell that sends out information) and the postsynaptic neuron (the cell that receives the information).

# U

**Unconscious mind**—Part of Freud's iceberg model, it contains all the things we are not aware of, including many things that Freud believed we can't bear to see, such as the memories and emotions associated with trauma.

# Who said nursing can't be fun?

We're the leading "dot calm" resource when you're feeling stressed.

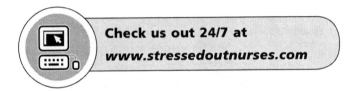

**Check us out 24/7 at**
***www.stressedoutnurses.com***

**What will you find there? Along with this colorful character, you'll see:**

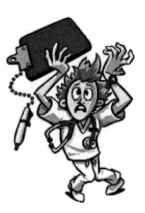

- ✔ **Contests**
- ✔ **Fun, witty articles that will help relieve your stress**
- ✔ **Resources to help you on your journey as a nurse**
- ✔ **Much, much more**

**So, what are you waiting for?**

**Get clicking and kiss your stress goodbye!**